A Touch *of* Hope

A Touch *of* Hope

A Hands-On Healer Shares the Miraculous Power of Touch

DEAN KRAFT

with Rochelle Kraft

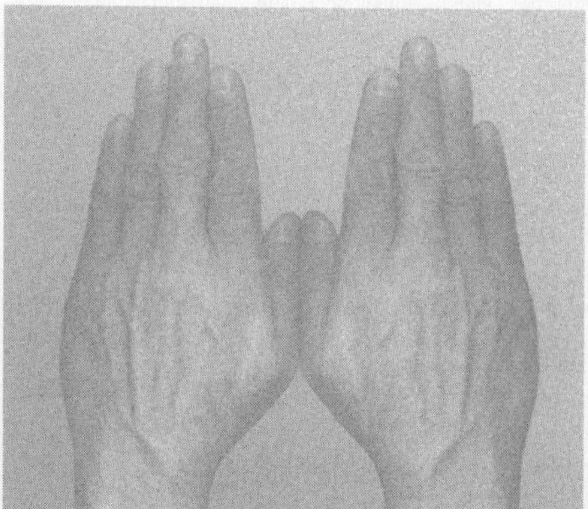

BERKLEY BOOKS, NEW YORK

A TOUCH OF HOPE

A Berkley Book / published by arrangement with
the authors

PRINTING HISTORY
G. P. Putnam's Sons edition / April 1998
Berkley trade paperback edition / July 1999

Text design by Deborah Kerner.
Illustrations by Jackie Aher.
Cover photo by Christine Rodin.

For information address:
The Berkley Publishing Group, a division of Penguin Putnam Inc.,
375 Hudson Street, New York, New York 10014.

The Penguin Putnam Inc. World Wide Web site address is
http://www.penguinputnam.com

ISBN: 0-425-16868-9

BERKLEY®
Berkley Books are published by
The Berkley Publishing Group, a division of Penguin Putnam Inc.,
375 Hudson Street, New York, New York 10014.
BERKLEY and the "B" design are trademarks
belonging to Penguin Putnam Inc.

PRINTED IN THE UNITED STATES OF AMERICA

10 9 8 7 6 5 4 3 2 1

Contents

Author's Note

This is a true story.
Some of the names have been changed
to protect private individuals
from any unwanted attention.

Acknowledgments

THIS BOOK IS NOT JUST ABOUT MY LIFE AS A HEALER, it is about two lives, for it includes that of my wife of twenty-two years, Rochelle, who has been my partner, constant companion, lover, and best friend. For almost thirty years she has been my anchor and an impartial observer of who I have been, what I have experienced, and who I have become. She has been the mirror of my soul and has brought order to the chaos of being a public person.

I will be forever grateful and indebted to Rochelle for her continual sacrifices, inspiration, remarkable writing skill, unselfishness, and, last but certainly not least, her undying love. If not for Rochelle, my dreams and those of many others I helped along the years never would have materialized. She is indeed the wind beneath my wings.

A very special thank-you to my mom and dad for their unconditional love and total acceptance of their unusual son. Also, to Rochelle's parents, Florence and David.

Rochelle and I both would like to express our deepest gratitude and appreciation to our editor, Nanscy Neiman-Legette, for her sensitive guidance and much-needed encouragement. Her keen insight and notable editorial prowess continually inspired us and kept us from straying from our mutual vision. We would also like to thank Marilyn Ducksworth and Michael Barson for helping us get this book to you, Jackie Aher for her beautiful illustrations, Hillery Borton for being there for us above and beyond the call of duty, and everyone at the Putnam Berkley Group who participated in making this book the best it can be.

Many thanks to our literary agents, Perry Knowlton, Andrew Pope, Timothy Knowlton, Ed Wintle, Dave Barbor, and to the rest of the team at Curtis Brown, Ltd.

And to all the people who have loved and shared with us through the good times and the difficult ones, we thank you from the bottoms of our hearts—you know who you are.

A Touch *of* Hope

I

A Normal Day

FOR THE FIRST TIME IN HOURS I ACTUALLY HEARD the soft classical music that wafted through my suite of offices as I took a few moments for myself. It had been a very busy morning, and as I glanced at my list of patients still to be seen, I realized that the rest of the day was going to be the same. *So many ill and desperate people,* I thought to myself as I scanned the piece of paper. And I wanted to give each person as much time as he or she needed, as much healing energy as I could, and as much hope as possible—no wonder I was running more than an hour behind. Normally I saw up to twenty people in a day, but my wife, Rochelle, had kept the day lighter because I had promised to fly to Chicago that night, after I was through in the office, for an emergency case.

The intercom between my office and Rochelle's buzzed, and she asked me if I was ready to see Marilyn. I told her to give me two more minutes and then send her in. We both blew little quiet kisses into the phone and hung up. After all these years, it made me feel good to know that Rochelle and I still had that special magic together.

I closed my eyes; took a few slow, deep breaths; cleared my mind of all the pain and sickness I'd already dealt with in the first half of my day; and prepared myself mentally for the next wave of patients. The people coming in needed me to be calm and focused.

As a laying-on-of-hands energy healer, I had tremendous responsibility and pressure resting on my shoulders. The people I saw in my brownstone office in Manhattan had been told by their doctors that nothing more could be done for them—and I was determined to try to help them anyway. It's not easy learning to live with constant pain, severe limitations, or the knowledge that you've got only months or weeks left to live. Many people had sought me out in a last, determined effort to change their doctors' dire prognoses. I became their guide, leading them through their fear and hopelessness and back onto a more optimistic road to better health. What a contrast to my initial reluctance to enter the field of alternative healing many years back.

Scanning my list again, I saw I had seven more patients to see—and I'd almost forgotten that Lucille Ball was due to come in for the first time. I wondered what she would be like and felt a little tingle of excitement—anticipation. Though celebrity clients were commonplace in my practice and added a bit of spice to the day, they also created more of a stir in the office and often took longer. I saw that Rochelle had prudently allowed more time than usual in my schedule for Lucy's first treatment—she probably assumed we could get to the airport at a reasonable time without rushing.

There was a gentle knock on my door, and Marilyn Englese walked in. We hugged, and as she sat at the edge of my plush leather massage table, she asked about me and then began to tell me how well she was doing. Marilyn was in her thirties, the attractive mother of two teenage girls and the wife of a school principal. As she shared with me the progress she'd experienced since her last session two months before, I thought back to the first time I saw her.

•

Marilyn had tried everything she could think of to escape the demons of her depression: transcendental meditation for three years, a psychiatrist for a year, and megavitamin therapy at the Nassau Mental Health Center for two years—all without success. She had lived in her private hell for seven years, had difficulty in caring for her family, and was beginning to believe that there was no help for her anywhere, until she'd heard about me through a friend.

The Marilyn I knew now was a warm, funny lady, ready to help someone else if she could, but you never would have known that in the beginning. Her desolation had altered her beyond recognition. She had been taking heavy doses of antidepressants but was eager to find a more natural way of getting help. Since she was already under the care of medical doctors, one of my prerequisites, I gave Marilyn an appointment.

The first time I saw her she was so sad that I was brought almost to tears. Fear and despair practically oozed from her, but it was her hazel eyes that silently spoke volumes about her desperation to break through the darkness of her melancholy. Immediately upon meeting her I felt I would be able to help her, but of course I did not tell her this—I had no idea how she would respond to my treatment or how long it could take. Each case was different—some people quickly reacted positively to my ministrations within just a session or two, others took longer, and some did not respond at all. I had not known which category Marilyn would fall into but hoped that she would give my form of energy treatment at least three to five attempts, to give us both a fair chance of altering her bleak state.

•

Looking up from my notes, I refocused on Marilyn and smiled at her. "Just remembering how far you've come, my dear," I said.

"I'm just so grateful to have found you, Dean," Marilyn said as she removed her shoes and stretched out on the table, ready for me to begin work. "And now that I only see you once in a while for maintenance, I appreciate what you've done for me even more."

I got up from my chair, walked the two steps to the table, and stood near her head. I closed my eyes, took a few calming breaths, and very lightly placed my hands around her head. The energy that flowed from my hands was automatic: it was like turning on a light switch; it was there, as always, on command. As I visualized and felt the smooth transference of energy entering her body, once again my thoughts drifted back through the years to Marilyn's initial sessions.

•

In the beginning it seemed questionable to me that Marilyn ever would respond the way I had believed she would—it was slow going. During the first few sessions, which were twice weekly, we focused on trying to break through her cycle of hopelessness and anxiety. Although she had been through so many other therapies without seeing any real change, I had confidence that I could help. Slowly, even through the haze of her medication, which I had insisted she remain on for the time being, she began to feel the same optimism. I hoped she would continue to respond positively.

I remember the feeling of my hands being guided to her head, then becoming very hot and giving off the usual vibratory sensation. Along with my mental image of balancing the chemicals in her brain, I had also visualized seeing her lively, happy, and healthy. This healing energy that flowed from my hands had relaxed her mind and body—the rigid tension she'd had was gone. Then I had concentrated on boosting her immune system.

After many weeks, the changes that had been subtle were now more obvious. After a few months of steady treatment, Marilyn came in renewed, describing how she had felt a heavy veil or curtain finally lift and disappear. She related feeling happiness for the first time in many years—and now she wanted to stop the antidepressants, which had never given her this joy. I had encouraged her to be patient and had suggested she see her doctor again, tell him about my intervention in her case, and then let him determine if it was appropriate to wean her off the medication.

My policy has always been for patients to inform their medical doctors that they are trying alternative healing methods, ones which create no conflict but rather work as complements to traditional Western medical avenues. Unfortunately there have been many cases where physicians who are skeptical about alternative healing or holistic medicine get so insulted at the mere mention of the idea that they immediately cut the patients off from their services, or threaten to do so if they continue. This creates fear and intimidation in so many patients that most never even attempt to tell their doctors that they are exploring complementary healing methods.

Marilyn was fortunate to have a doctor who was open-minded enough to acknowledge her relatively sudden positive changes. He had agreed to begin to lower the medication she so dreaded, and within weeks Marilyn was medication-free, doing better than ever, and had begun to focus on a new life without the burden of severe depression.

•

I shook myself and came back to the present. I continued working with Marilyn, moving my hands above her heart region and back to her head and neck, then once again gently touching her shoulders until I felt the treatment was complete. I glanced at my watch and saw that twenty minutes had flown by.

I lowered my arms and hands to my sides, took in and released a few deep breaths, and instructed Marilyn to do the same. She knew it was the end of her session and, like most everyone, was reluctant to get up from the table. Finally she raised herself up on an elbow and smiled at me. This was what it was all about—helping people.

Slowly she gathered her shoes and handbag and, enjoying her pleasant after-treatment glow, gave me a big hug.

"Dean, I just can't thank you enough for giving me my life back," Marilyn said as she made her way out of my office to schedule her next appointment with Rochelle.

There was no time for any more reflection as I checked my list to see who was due next. I was still behind schedule and had to get moving. Rochelle came into my office, closed the door, and told me she'd ordered some sandwiches to be delivered when she'd realized we would not be able to get out for lunch. I asked if I had time to see Jonathan before the food arrived. She said I did and, after a quick kiss, she left.

Within moments there was a knock on my door and Rochelle led in my next patient, Jonathan Felt. He was a friendly guy in his late twenties who was currently a producer for the ABC documentary program "20/20." We shook hands. As he proped his lean athletic form against the side of the massage table, I could tell he was excited about something. I guess the huge grin on his face was my first clue.

"Dean, do you remember what my leg looked like two weeks ago?"

"Of course I do," I responded as I sat down at my desk, retrieved his file from the stack, and got ready to make follow-up notations for his third session.

"Well, wait 'til you see it now!" he said eagerly as he lifted his leg onto the table and began to peel back the bandages. "You're not going to believe it!"

Jonathan had been in an automobile accident nine years earlier and had undergone repeated operations throughout those years in an attempt to close a gaping hole in his shin. There had been some success, but it had never healed completely. After three years of conventional treatment, the one-inch open wound in his shin still simply refused to mend. Despite every available traditional option, including plastic surgery, the injury remained the same. Then Jonathan read an article about my work and came to see me.

During our first session together, Jonathan had been skeptical and had confessed his doubtfulness in my type of treatment being able to help him, but he had quickly added that at this point he was willing to try anything. I had explained that his *belief* in alternative healing was unnecessary, that all that was needed for us to work together was his *willingness* to give it a try. As usual, I promised nothing, other than that I would do the best I could to try to stimulate his own healing system to complete the job the surgeries could not.

Then I saw the wound. It was a raw, gaping hole, and the surrounding skin was swollen and angry-looking dark red—not a pretty sight. I felt a bit queasy—I really did not like to see such graphic injuries.

Now, just one month later, he was enthusiastic to show me the changes. The beginnings of the healing were obvious. There was now only a tiny pinhead of an opening, and the skin was flatter, smoother, and paler, more natural-looking.

"And how's the pain been?" I asked him, making quick notes in his file.

"Much better, actually almost gone completely. And I don't limp anymore, either. I think this is pretty incredible, don't you?"

And before I could agree, he told me more about a new program he was producing for the documentary series, sharing some of his life with me. Then he said that since he'd gotten relief from me that his medical doctors could not give him, he was very interested in doing a piece on "20/20" featuring my work. Apparently, his opinion about this form of healing had changed dramatically with his firsthand experience. Naturally, my interest was piqued. Sharing my ideas in a national forum was always appealing and important, but by this time I had gotten so much media attention that I knew the end results—I would be further deluged with a fresh outpouring of people seeking my help. Because my patients also usually referred friends or relatives to me, my practice was already pushing out at the seams.

"Thanks, Jonathan," I replied, "but I don't think so. I really don't want to disappoint a lot of people who won't be able to get in to me. I already have a long waiting list, and my schedule is just too jam-packed.

But thanks for asking—I appreciate the invitation and especially your change in attitude."

Jonathan could not argue with this—he had always seen my waiting room full—so finally he stretched his long body down onto the table. I asked him to close his eyes, take a few slow deep breaths, and clear his mind of work. I wanted him to relax so that his body would be primed to receive my ministrations.

I switched on the portable fan that sat on my desk, and its steady drone helped me quiet myself, blocking out the murmuring voices in the waiting room and the noises of the city. After a few moments, I stood up and positioned myself next to the table near Jonathan's shin. I held both of my hands around his lower leg, encircling the wounded area but not touching it, and visualized a thick white band of healing light entering it. In my mind I "saw" the hole closing completely, fully healed. I was completely confident that if I could stimulate Jonathan's natural healing system, his body would then take over and complete its inborn function—healing the wound. After a few minutes of concentrating on this image, I felt my hands generating great heat. Right at that moment, Jonathan opened his eyes and looked at my hands. He saw I was not touching him and voiced his amazement over the unusual warmth he felt, not only around the injury but throughout his whole body. Softly, Jonathan whispered, "Dean, that feels so soothing, so calming."

I then moved to the opposite end of the table and very gently layed both my hands on his temples, then his head and neck. Jonathan commented on the unusual vibrations coming from my hands and fingers.

Again time flew by and the session was over. I told him to take a few deep breaths before sitting up, and then said, "I'm beginning to teach more of my patients mental self-help exercises to do at home. Would you like to learn a visualization technique you could practice in between our treatments?"

"You bet! I'd love to," he answered intently.

I told him to lie down again, eyes closed. He was already very relaxed, so I described what I wanted him to "see" in his mind. I instructed him to invent a thick white band of warm healing light that was an inch or two wide, traveling around the outside of his body, and then reaching the area of his injury. I encouraged him to use his mind to see the band of light expanding, surrounding, and entering the wound. In addition, I told him to visualize the hole in his leg becoming smaller and smaller until it was completely closed.

We spent about ten minutes reviewing this over and over until he said he felt confident that he understood. I urged him to do this at home at least once a day, relaxing himself for a few minutes first so he could focus entirely on the various aspects.

As he prepared to leave, he gave me a quick hug and thanked me.

"Think about it, Dean. If you change your mind, I'd love to do a piece on you."

I smiled affirmatively and told him to check his schedule and rebook with Rochelle, and then made some final notes about his remarkable recovery.

After taking a few deep gulps of water, I walked through the reception area, greeting the patients waiting, and headed for the small bathroom to wash my hands and face. As I walked back to my office, Rochelle stopped me, handed me a new-patient form, and told me Lucille Ball, the next to be seen, was waiting outside in her block-long limousine. It seemed she was attracting quite a crowd, for the limo had a license plate that read "I ♥ Lucy" and strangers were waving to her and trying to peek inside past the darkened windows. Lunch would have to wait. I told Rochelle to bring her in and, as I walked back to my office, I reviewed the record sheet she'd handed me. Arthritis. Easy stuff, I thought to myself.

Opening my door a minute later, Rochelle led in the refined and casually dressed red-haired comedian, indicated a chair for her to sit in, and closed the door quietly. The fresh cold air lingered on Lucy, and it was like a tonic in my sweltering office. We smiled at each other, and I had to strain my neck way back in order to look into her eyes—she was very tall and towered over me. We shook hands, and then she sat down and came right to the point.

"Dean, I'm here because I was very impressed with what you did for a close friend of mine, Paula."

I nodded, indicating I knew whom she was talking about—a woman with cervical cancer who'd come to see me the year before.

"Well, she can't say enough wonderful things about you," Lucy said, and went on to explain that she was in New York temporarily to film a movie, portraying a bag lady in an upcoming television drama. She was anxious to know whether I could help her in the brief time she'd be in town.

"Lucy, relax. Let's take it a step at a time. Tell me more about your problem."

"The arthritis is in my knees, ankles, wrists, and hands. It's been bad for years but it's really acting up—and I have to finish this movie!" Realizing she was a bit frantic, she sighed, settled back in her chair, and said, "Look, I realize my problem isn't life-threatening, like Paula's was, but it's still making it very hard for me to work."

I began making notations and asked her to rate the pain from one to ten, ten being the worst.

"Right now it's so bad I'd have to say it's a ten. All of my joints are stiff and hurt like hell."

"When did you see a doctor last, and what did he do for you?" I asked, still scribbing as I spoke.

"Just yesterday, and he probed my knees and wrists so hard that it made me want to scream! Then he suggested giving me a steroid injection but I told him those shots hurt so bad—no, thank you. Besides, they only help for a while and I've already had so many of them. They're not good for your liver, you know. So what do you think, can you help me, or what?" she nearly shouted.

"Well, I can't promise you anything, but let's give it a try. In my experience, arthritis doesn't usually require long-term treatment. Hopefully a few sessions close together could make a difference, so let's see how it goes."

I questioned her about any other health problems she had, and then, after talking about fifteen minutes, I asked her to move over to the table, remove her shoes, and stretch out. She was having a problem bending, so I helped remove her shoes. She took off her large clip-on earrings, put them on the side of my desk, and awkwardly got onto the table. After placing the pillow I handed to her under her knees, she squirmed about until she was comfortable, or as comfortable as she could get, under the circumstances. A whiff of her perfume floated through the room, and I recognized it as something Rochelle sometimes wore. I complimented her on her scent, and she began telling me about where she'd bought it, but I was already preparing to work. Her voice was a background buzz.

Within a few moments and several breaths in and out to clear my mind and relax, I asked Lucy to close her eyes, too.

"Just breathe normally and let me know if you need another pillow under your knees," I said.

"It feels perfect," she answered.

"I'm just going to try and act as a catalyst to your own healing system, kind of like charging up your battery so that it's rejuvenated and can work on its own," I said.

"Fine with me," she responded. "Charge away!"

Standing at the head of the table, I began by lightly placing both my palms on her temples. After a minute, I lifted my hands and held them about six inches above her head. In my mind I saw her stiff knee and ankle joints welded together, unmovable, and then imagined them transforming before my eyes, becoming more fluid and moving with ease. As I moved to the side of the table and touched her wrists, I could sense that the energy I was emitting flowed smoothly. I could also tell she was already relaxing and enjoying the experience.

"Jeez," she said suddenly, "your hands are burning hot!"

"Is it uncomfortable?" I queried.

"Not at all—it feels terrific!" she said quietly.

Systematically and with awareness that she was in pain, I lightly placed my hands on and over the various problem areas and visualized the stiff calcium deposits and spindicles shrinking, dissolving, and then disappearing.

About twenty minutes later, I felt our first session together had gone well and in a tranquil tone told Lucy to take a few deep breaths and open her eyes. She didn't move, and at first I thought she'd fallen into a light sleep, for her breathing was soft and steady. I wasn't surprised—that happens fairly frequently when someone finally lets go and relaxes. I gave her another minute and again told her she could open her eyes.

"That was unbelievable!" she said as she tried to shake herself out of her haze. "I can't remember being so relaxed! Hey, Dean, can we bottle this stuff?" She let out a loud cackle, and I couldn't help laughing myself. I said, "I'd like to bottle that laugh!" and we shared the beginnings of a bonding that is so important in this type of work. Yes, it had gone well.

She sat up and swung her legs more easily onto the floor, still looking a bit dazed.

I sat down on the chair by my desk and smiled at her. I said, "Okay, if you'd like, you can schedule another session later this week with Rochelle, and we'll take it one step at a time." After working with people in this unusual manner for years now, I'd learned not to ask if someone was feeling better immediately afterward—I knew they'd tell me.

As if reading my mind Lucy offered, "The pain is so much better, it's almost hard to believe." I made a note that before she left she was able to put her shoes on by herself. Then, at the same time, we extended our arms to each other for a hug before she slowly made her way out to see Rochelle.

I began to straighten the room for the next person, changing the pillow cases and the paper on the table. Suddenly I noticed something sparkling on my desk—Lucy's earrings. Shaking my head and grinning,

I grabbed them and rushed out of my room to return them, and saw Lucy, eyes still glazed over, heading toward me. I dropped the gold disks into her hands, and we both giggled.

"Ya know, you made me feel so good I could've left my head on that table and walked out if it wasn't attached. 'Bye!"

I needed to take a break, so I chatted with the people in the waiting room for a few moments. They were all abuzz about seeing Lucy in the office.

Finally I was able to chomp down a tuna sandwich before the rest of the day sped by.

The last person I had to see was Marcy Goldstein, a medical doctor and acupuncturist. He was in his late fifties, a generation older than I. We had met a number of years before, when he'd sought my help in Florida, where I was living at the time. Since then, he had recommended a number of patients and was so impressed with their positive reactions that he subsequently had me treat many of his own unresponsive patients in his office, while overseeing and documenting their changes. Over the years, Marcy has observed countless unexplainable and miraculous recoveries through my treatments.

Recently we had been working together on a much more serious problem—Marcy had been diagnosed with an unusual glomus tumor in his neck, pressing dangerously against the jugular vein. It was creating hearing loss and tinnitus, a ringing in his head that was synchronous with his pulse. A traditionally trained medical doctor, he took all the proper medical steps in order to get a thorough diagnosis. He was extremely concerned with the results. After his condition had been determined, he immediately came to see me again.

If I was unable to shrink or dissolve this mass that was starting to acutely constrict his jugular, he would have to endure very complicated and risky surgery, possibly creating other complications. He was willing to undergo this surgery only if my methods failed. I treated him intensively for ten days, trying to recede the tumor, and hoped that he would not require the possibly life-threatening surgery usually required in cases such as his.

Marcy was not just one of the many doctors I worked with professionally. He and his wife, Miriam, had become good friends of Rochelle's and mine, so I was especially nervous for him—I wanted our treatments together to be fruitful and hoped I had at least begun the process of slowing or stopping this progressive and dangerous growth.

The intercom buzzed, and Rochelle told me that Marcy was on his way in. Almost six feet tall with a full graying beard and round wire-rimmed glasses, Marcy was beaming with a smile that spread from ear to ear. He gave me a huge hug that almost lifted me off the floor.

"You did it!" he hollered. "You really did it!"

Excitedly he pulled out X rays and, one by one, held them above the lamp on my desk. He pointed out where the tumor had been, and then got the original X rays and showed me the difference. The tumor seemed to have disappeared completely, and although the doctors had no explanation for it and were thoroughly confused, Marcy and I were beyond delighted.

We both jumped up and down like two kids, slapping each other's hands in a high-five—it was terrific to be able to do this work, but it was especially satisfying to help a friend.

I started to tell Marcy a little about the case I was about to take on: a little girl in Chicago had almost drowned and had been in a coma for six weeks, with no signs of coming out of it. I recalled how desperately the child's mother had pleaded with me to help her daughter.

Within minutes of saying good-bye to an elated Marcy, Rochelle and I were off to the airport to try to create another unexplainable recovery. The taxi sped through the cold and darkened streets of Manhattan.

It had been a long day, even with the lighter schedule. I felt exhausted, and I wasn't finished yet.

Because of New York's late rush-hour traffic, plane delays, and bumper-to-bumper tie-ups in the Windy City, it was almost midnight as Rochelle and I hurried toward Children's Hospital. The overdue hour didn't matter, the child's mother had said when Rochelle phoned from the airport to explain our lateness. Time was of the essence for five-year-old Jessica, who had fallen into Lake Michigan. The young child had been trapped under the frozen ice for a very long period before finally being rescued. Now her life-support systems were about to be turned off.

A pretty young woman with dark hair was standing outside the hospital with her arms wrapped around herself, trying to keep out the raw, wintry air. As Rochelle and I left the warmth of the taxi, the frigid wind blasted me in the face and actually revived me. The little girl's mother, Suzanne, was barely controlling her hysteria as she led us from the taxi to a side entrance she used after visiting hours. We walked through the deserted hallways, speaking very softly about her daughter. Our footsteps echoed solemnly in the silence as we made our way to the elevator that would take us to the Intensive Care floor. As we waited, Suzanne kept wringing her hands with anxiety. I placed a hand lightly on her shoulder, looked into her anguished eyes, and said reassuringly that I would do everything in my power to try to bring her child out of the coma.

Suzanne led us into the Intensive Care room, and I saw a small motionless form laying in a bed, tubes connected to her nose, throat, and arms. There were various beeping sounds and a conglomerate of machinery around her, including a respirator, which enabled her to live in the dormant state. She was a miniature of her mother, slightly built, with the same straight brown hair and high cheek bones. Her eyes were closed, and her breathing was shallow and mechanical. One of the monitors displayed her EEG brain-wave pattern, and I was dismayed when I saw there were no wavy lines—it was flat, lifeless, just like Jessica appeared.

The antiseptic odor assaulted my nose, and unconsciously I began to breathe through my mouth. The room was full of curious doctors and nurses who were all privy to what I was about to attempt. In these types of severe cases, the attending medical staff always had to give permission for my intervention. I sought out one of the doctors in charge at the time, and learned that they considered Jessica hopeless, brain dead. Because her condition was steadily deteriorating since her belated rescue, they felt their only remaining course of action was to discontinue all forms of artificial life support and allow her to die naturally.

I had other plans for Jessica.

For some unknown reason, I am able to "will" myself to join people in the strange ether of a coma. This was not the first time I was going to try to bring someone back from the tight grip of that dimension, but still it was very risky. Rochelle was aware of the potential hazards of my doing this, but understood why I had to try.

I knew the doctors and nurses had to remain, but I persuaded Suzanne to sit outside the room with Rochelle. As Rochelle was leading her out, Suzanne turned back and grabbed my hand, her eyes brimming with tears. I could hear her silent plea.

I wrapped my fingers around hers, smiled encouragingly, and said, "Don't give up, Suzanne, don't ever give up hope."

I walked back into the room and pulled up a chair near the bed, and closed my eyes. It took a few minutes for me to totally blank out the curious staring faces, the sounds of machines ticking and beeping, and the palpable tension in the room.

Then I lifted a tiny doll-like hand and spoke forcefully: "Jessica . . . I'm Dean . . . a friend. Your mom brought me here to try to help you get better. If you hear me, I want you to squeeze my hand."

I repeated this several times and kept waiting to feel even the slightest bit of returned pressure on my hand, but there was no response. I knew then that this one was not going to be easy.

I pushed back the chair and stood at the head of her bed. With Jessica's hand still in mine, I tenderly placed my other hand on her forehead. My thoughts were completely focused on stimulating and resuscitating her life force, but I received no energylike sonar feedback. Again, this was an indication that I had to try even harder.

Relax, Dean, I said to myself. *Just calm down and try to connect.* Within moments I felt I was no longer in the hospital room but being swept away with a sudden rush of wind, propelled through a tunnel-like tube, sucked along and tumbling through this shaft of pipeline. I sensed rather than saw swirling patterns of brilliant lights. No longer bounded by my physical body, my entire essence was like a floating conscious mind that was quickly pulsating with the sounds of my heartbeat.

Hurling through these lights and wind gusts at tremendous speed, I suddenly realized that everything had become very silent and still. All I could see was a fog, a haze. Then, far off in the blackness, I saw a faint bluish-white glow, which I believed was Jessica's lightform.

Silently I called out, "Jessica, I'm here to bring you back to your mother. Jessica, answer me."

Silence. I waited patiently. When I noiselessly called to her again, I thought I heard a faint childish voice.

"I'm scared," I heard. "Where am I? Mommy!"

"Don't be scared, honey, I'm here to bring you home to Mommy. She sent me to get you, so there's nothing to be frightened of. . . ."

I felt myself moving closer to the weak glow of her lightbody, and as I wafted closer I could hear her whimpering. In a flash, my own lightbody enveloped hers and I felt like a lifeguard struggling through a sudden raging squall, fighting off the forces that seemed to want to pull Jessica from my grasp.

I feared we weren't going to make it, when the next thing I knew I was back in the hospital room, the bright overhead lights blinding me, my body slumped in the chair, my hand still tightly gripping Jessica's. Now, out of my altered state, I saw Jessica's body jerk a few times and then relax. Slowly I became more aware of the room. There was a stampede of activity: machines started sounding off loudly, and as a flurry of bodies moved around me, someone handed me a glass of water. I downed the liquid and held out the tumbler for more.

Two doctors and the head nurse surrounded me, all hammering me with questions at the same time:

"What did you do?"

"What happened?"

"Are you all right?"

"What the hell is going on here?"

Without answering, I looked at the EEG monitor by the bed and saw small wavy lines rhythmically cross the screen.

It indicated life.

I was elated as I tried to refocus on the questions that were pummeling me now from all directions. The medical staff concentrated on their tasks of monitoring the machines and examining Jessica, faces alight with disbelief and amazement instead of desperation and hopelessness.

I kept staring at Jessica. As her small body shifted in tiny movements around the bed, her eyes opened, and, in spite of the respirator tube in her throat, her attempts to talk were obvious as she mouthed the words, "Mommy . . . Mommy."

Pandemonium continued as a few still-frozen nurses began rushing about attending to their newly revived patient. Several had tissues pressed against their eyes. Finally I began to answer the doctors but realized I was exhausted.

Suzanne rushed into the room and lay herself on the bed, cradling her child and whispering loving words into her ear. I just sat and watched as Suzanne finally got off the bed, came over to me, and threw her arms around me, crying. Gratefully she realized how drained I was and she suggested that we talk about the miraculous events the following day, when things hopefully would be settled down.

When I felt stronger and was ready to leave, I spoke with the doctors in charge and promised to get them some of my documentation—published articles about my work, and testimonials from patients, doctors, and scientists—to help explain my unusual occupation. I turned around and walked back to Jessica, who was whimpering and snuggling close to her mother. Affectionately, I kissed her on her forehead, and my reward was a smile from the little girl—a knowing smile.

Rochelle held on to me as we left the hospital and got into a taxi that seemed to be waiting just for us. With instructions to take us to O'Hare

Airport, the taxi sped off. When the cab entered a tunnel toward the airport, the bright lights sped by hypnotically. I stared at them in a weary daze and I thought back to the beginning—when I was coming out of another tunnel just like it in Brooklyn, New York, when I was just a normal guy. . . .

2

My Strange Path *to* Healing

It was late autumn, November 22, 1972. The date is forever emblazoned in my mind. My boss, Buddy, and I lived near each other in Brooklyn, New York, so we made a habit of driving home together after closing the music store. We were in his leased 1971 beige Buick Electra, a luxurious car, and the soft brown leather bench seat felt great after a hectic day in Manhattan.

We had been rehashing the day's business events, and Buddy had just turned from the Prospect Expressway tunnel onto Ocean Parkway, when all four electric door locks in the car began clicking rapidly up and down. After making sure that neither of us was touching the control panel buttons, Buddy and I naturally concluded that the locks clicking on their own were the result of an electrical short. But this had never happened before, and the locks continued to move up and down every couple of minutes, unprovoked by either of us. Buddy was annoyed because now he would have to make the time to bring the car to a garage for repairs.

Then, jokingly, Buddy suggested perhaps some "spirit" was responsible for the locks moving and maybe his deceased mother was trying to communicate with him.

Joining in his game, I dramatically commanded, "If there is a spirit in this car, give me five clicks!"

Click. . . . Click. . . . Click. . . . Click. . . . Click.

We stared at each other, aghast, and laughed out loud. What an incredible coincidence! Then we called for more clicks from the car. Sure, we felt pretty dumb, talking to his car, but the loose wire or whatever was making the door locks move responded correctly to commands for ten and then fifteen clicks.

This was no longer funny. Trying to come up with some rational explanation, Buddy pulled the car off to the side of the road and turned the engine off, figuring that the door locks would stop moving since they were electrical. Neither of us quite believed that the other wasn't playing some kind of joke, so, to be sure, we sat in the middle of the seat, held each other's hands, and wrapped our legs across each other. I smiled and was just contemplating the possibility of a policeman spotting us like that—"Oh, hi, officer, we're just communing with spirits"—when Buddy quietly asked, "How much is two plus two?"

Four jumps of the locks immediately answered. Then silence.

This was no coincidence. It was impossible, yet it was happening. Initially I was convinced that Buddy had to be playing a trick on me. But when I saw his expression, I had to dismiss the idea. The hair at the nape of his neck was literally curling up. By this time, I'd known Buddy for several years and in all sorts of situations, even during attempted armed robberies at the store, but I had never seen him look so frightened.

We were quiet as we continued home, each of us immersed in his own thoughts. When I stepped out of the car that night, I felt anxious, chilled, confused, and covered with goose bumps. I was scared, but didn't know of what. There was this weird "feeling" in the car. . . .

Later that night, Buddy called me to say that the door locks had stopped moving after he dropped me off and he was very disappointed.

And he was adamant that it all had something to do with me. After I hung up with Buddy, I sat back, with my head resting on the couch, stared at the bright light fixture overhead, and closed my eyes. My head began to swim. It was not a glitch in the electrical system—there was something very strange going on. This I felt sure of, and deep inside, although I resisted what Buddy said, I knew it had something to do with me. . . .

Why me?

Growing up in a middle-class nontraditional Jewish family, I wasn't exposed to any particularly strong religious beliefs and my life was void of any psychic or supernatural encounters. I was never the least bit interested in anything related to the paranormal. Always very skeptical, logical, and scientific by nature, I was generally curious about how things worked. I never read any books or studied anything to do with psychics or mystical or esoteric subjects.

On the whole, I felt I had an unremarkable childhood. My parents had met during World War II in Washington, D.C.—my father had just joined the Army, and my mother was a clerical worker. After the war, they lived in New York until a job for my father drew them back to Washington in 1950. On April 14 of that year, I was born. Shortly thereafter, my father's independent nature asserted itself and he opened a small grocery store, Tiny's Market, named for my mother, who's less than five feet tall.

When I was seven years old, I had what I consider my first unusual experience.

I recall that I was wearing only a thin jacket over my clothes, for it was a warm spring day, kicking a soccer ball way across the schoolyard. The ball dropped down into a steep stairwell that led to the school basement. As I ran to get it, a friend called out to me, diverting my attention, and the next thing I knew, I had stumbled over the ledge of the stairwell. In what felt like slow motion, I tumbled head over heels in the air, falling one full story to the hard pavement below.

Automatically, I covered my head protectively to soften the impending collision. Then, it was as if someone's broad hands cradled my head and body, gently lowering me onto the concrete. I was stunned for a moment, and then I jumped to my feet. I expected to see the teacher that had broken my fall, and I wanted to thank him or her, but there was no one there! I remember having goose bumps as big as quarters all over! Something very odd had just happened—I should have crushed my skull or, at the very least, bumped and scraped myself. But I did not have a scratch or bruise of any kind. This was the first conscious moment in my life when I felt someone or something was watching over me. It was eerie, but I quickly forgot about it until a couple of weeks later.

It was Passover time, and, though we were not religious, my parents, my older sister, Roberta, and my younger one, Lisa, and I still enjoyed having a special dinner, even reserving the traditional empty seat and place setting for Elijah. Right after Dad recited a prayer, the front door suddenly blew open on the still and windless night. We all were startled and we looked toward the door, but no one was there.

Mystified, Mom got up and closed the door, and when she returned to the table, we saw that Elijah's wineglass, which had been full a moment ago, was now half empty. The room was very quiet, then everyone talked at once about the chills that ran through us all. No one had touched the wine, and all the other glasses were still full. We sat there, staring at one another, and tried to make sense of it. Afterward, we decided that we had just had an unexpected visit from Elijah, and he was nice enough to show his presence by drinking some of the refreshment we had poured especially for him. It remains a family mystery.

By 1959, the family business was well established but the pain caused by my father's old Army injury grew severe, and his illness, with its grim prognosis of complete immobility, was identified. My folks sold the grocery and our house at a great loss, and we moved back to New York and into a one-bedroom apartment in Sheepshead Bay, Brooklyn. Dad's promised insurance-salesman position fell through, so he took three different delivery jobs to support the family until a better situation opened up, managing a small cosmetics firm in Williamsburg.

At thirteen I started working and bought myself an electric guitar. Not yet able to afford the amplifier, with a little experimentation and ingenuity, I turned an old broken phonograph into a good substitute. I taught myself to play, and in time I became proficient enough to play lead guitar and form my own rock group, which entertained at local dances and clubs.

In 1968 I took a part-time job as a music salesman at Buddy's Music, owned by Buddy Geier, which was on Quentin Road off Kings Highway, a popular shopping district in Brooklyn. A short, pleasant, and happy-go-lucky musician in his mid-fifties, Buddy had played saxophone for such well-loved leaders as Benny Goodman and Vaughn Monroe during the days of the Big Bands. From the first day he and I met, we really hit it off. Despite the difference in our ages, we had a great deal in common, and there was enough of a physical resemblance between us that we were often mistaken for father and son.

At Buddy's I quickly learned to play many different instruments because I had to demonstrate them for customers. Rock groups were forever in and out of the store, trading equipment and bits of gossip. We discussed groups, dates, performances—everything in the music field. I was finally in my element.

Within a couple of years, Buddy opened a second store on West Forty-eighth Street and Seventh Avenue in Manhattan, an area crowded with music stores and commonly referred to as the Music District. Buddy named me manager, and I knew then that my direction was music. Just before I turned twenty-one and after three full years and a 3.0 average, I decided to give up academia and withdrew from Long Island University. Who had the time anymore? I knew what I was going to do with my life. But now, almost two years later . . .

I was startled out of my daydream as my parents walked into the den. I decided not to tell them about the supernatural event that had just occurred in Buddy's car. I was afraid that they would commit me!

I figured I needed an objective third party in Buddy's car, so I called my friend and fellow musician, Sam Sunshine, who worked at a music store near Buddy's in the city. We made arrangements to meet in front of Buddy's at closing time the following day.

And the day dragged—I couldn't wait to get back into the car. Finally, we all piled into the Buick, and Buddy, Sam, and I began posing simple mathematical questions. Again, the door locks clicked the correct responses. Sam, a quiet, calm, and stable presence, checked all around us in the car and convinced himself that there were no tricks being played between me and Buddy. He was as fascinated as we were by not only the clicking door locks and the accurate answers to our commands, but also the tangibly mysterious atmosphere that pervaded.

Within a couple of days, Buddy brought his car in to be checked and was told by two different repair shops that there was nothing wrong with the electrical system. There were no loose wires or shorts of any kind. The car was in good working order. In weeks to come, Buddy's wife, Shirley, and at least ten other friends and acquaintances witnessed the eerie clicking of the door locks.

But they occurred only when I was in the car!

Each time I was about to tell my family, I thought twice and did not. It was all too insane. I hardly believed what was happening myself, yet the clicking door locks had happened so often in front of so many supposedly sane, reputable people that we had to rule out deception and mass hysteria. If it hadn't been for all the witnesses, I probably would have committed Buddy and myself for psychiatric evaluation.

Soon our liaison with the door locks grew more complex. First we developed a "one click for 'No,' two clicks for 'Yes' " code that enabled us to ask simple and often silly questions, like "Did we have a good day at the store today?"—questions we already knew the answers to. We constantly tested "it," and the responding 'Yes' or 'No' answers were always correct. Then we posed some in-depth, serious questions.

•

"Are you Buddy's deceased mother?"

Click.

"Are you from this planet?"

Click.

"Are you on a planet our scientists know of?"

Click.

"Another galaxy?"

Click, click.

"Are you all-knowing?"

Click, click.

"Are you over a thousand years old?"

Click, click.

•

To say we were astounded would have been quite an understatement.

Then we worked out an alphabet system: I would ask a question, and Buddy would slowly recite the alphabet, stopping whenever we heard a distinctive click. Sam became a regular fixture in the backseat and was armed with a pencil and some paper lying around (usually one of the dozens of bank receipts that cluttered the floor of Buddy's car). He would diligently write down the letter indicated by the click of the door locks. Then Buddy would start again from A until we heard another click. Individual letters formed words and sentences. Provided with this new verbal ability, the locks clicked out messages that ranged from the mundane to the seemingly prophetic.

Once, when Buddy and his wife, Shirley, were quarreling, we deciphered the words, SAUL THERE IS NO TIME FOR ARGUING YOU TWO WORRY TOO MUCH.

"Who the hell is Saul?" I asked.

Buddy turned ashen as he said, "Me. I'm Saul. That's my real name, but I never use it." I hadn't known that.

I kept up my attempt to carry on a normal existence, but it was becoming increasingly difficult, especially in front of my family. Still, every time I thought about the outrageousness of our sessions in the car, I erased the possibility of telling them. I was very preoccupied with the car and what it all could mean. It was impossible for anyone to experience this car phenomenon and not get obsessed with it.

Four weeks from our first "communication" in the car, a few days before Christmas 1972, I was working at Buddy's Music in Manhattan, when I heard the screech of a car, followed by agonized screams. I ran to the display window and watched in horror as a young woman, pinned under the low running board of an old car, was dragged down the street. I immediately ran out to help lift the car and free her.

The woman was bleeding profusely and seemed to be in shock. Without thinking, I knelt in the crowded street to try to comfort her, gently stroking the hair on her damp forehead. I saw Buddy standing back and watching just outside the store, and I yelled to him to bring me a blanket or something. I took the old drape he retrieved and gently placed it under her head to cushion it from the hard, winter street. I continued to stroke her forehead.

Suddenly, I experienced a strong, compassionate sensation—I perceived a connection, a "oneness" with this stranger that I'd never felt before. But before I could think further about it, an ambulance arrived and the attendants quickly removed the injured woman on a special slat stretcher, for their speedy diagnosis indicated broken bones. I could think of little else the rest of the day and felt more emotional than I ever remember. I actually cared about this unknown person in the street.

That night, as Buddy and I headed home in his car, I kept discussing the terrible incident with him, over and over again, when the door locks began clicking. We quickly learned that when "it" wanted to "talk," the locks would click up and down very rapidly to get our attention. It sure did—it would have gotten anyone's attention! But no longer quite as shocked at the things that happened in that car, I grabbed a pen and a scrap of paper from the littered floor as Buddy slowly began reciting the alphabet. The message read: DEAN YOUR HAND HEALED TODAY.

Immediately I looked at my hands for a cut or scratch that might have healed, but I saw nothing unusual and couldn't remember hurting myself. The locks clicked on.

HELP THOSE WHO NEED HELP.

It was Buddy that shakingly suggested that perhaps the healing the first message had referred to was connected with the car accident earlier in the day.

The idea seemed preposterous to me.

The following day, Buddy was irritable and complained that I was too wrapped up with this woman.

"Why do you care so much about her?" he asked.

Why *did* I? She was a stranger to me, yet I was compelled to call the hospital, which further incensed Buddy, since I used the store phone. I learned that the woman admitted to the hospital after the car accident on West Forty-eighth Street and Seventh Avenue the day before had been released with minor cuts and bruises.

The thought that I might have had anything to do with it was absurd, and I thoroughly rejected the ridiculous possibility. I looked down at my hands once again—there was nothing striking or remarkable about them—and dismissed the thought of strange healing powers. Let's be honest—I knew that the woman could have been misdiagnosed by the ambulance attendants on the scene. It had nothing to do with me at all, but I was happy the lady was all right.

Yet my life continued on its unusual voyage. One evening, Buddy, Sam, and I were having dinner together at a restaurant in downtown Manhattan before going home. We frequently postponed the end of the evening to savor the experience of what we knew would come with our new "friend." Buddy was happily telling Sam and me about this new mind-control course he was taking, and was expounding on things I'd never heard of before, when his voice slowly faded and a loud *hhuuumm-mmmm* filled my ears. I abruptly felt nauseous and dizzy. Buddy and Sam were quite concerned because, they said, I looked terrible. I couldn't speak. I sat in a stupor, staring intently at the giant wood-block table at which we were sitting.

I began to feel a tingling all over. Flashes of heat raced through my body. A pounding in my temples began, like a hammer beating some foreign tune. I found it hard to draw a full breath and I was terrified! Could I be having a heart attack at twenty-two? Honestly, at this stage it would not have surprised me.

Then I had a vision. I saw myself, as if from a distance, stretched out on the floor of the restaurant, on my stomach, and the base of the large table we were sitting at was on top of my back! I could actually feel the pressure on my spine, and tried to shake it off.

I felt as though my brain were pulsating, I was hyperventilating, and with every exertion of breath, it seemed as though my head were expanding. Then I felt a sudden sharp pinprick in the center of my forehead, and what seemed to be compressed power or energy that had built up inside me began to pour out. It flowed to my vision of the table on my back. Abruptly, the *actual* table in front of us started moving, rattling the glasses and dishes. Buddy and Sam jumped away and raised the tablecloth. They saw that no part of my body was touching the table. I was still sitting, motionless, staring blankly, when I felt myself grow faint. The pounding in my temples ceased, my breathing slowed, my head dropped to my chest, and the table stopped moving.

I felt dreadfully ill, but refused offers of assistance as I slowly made my way to the bathroom to splash cold water on my face and neck. That made me feel a little better, but an odd sensation remained. Still dazed, I rejoined Buddy and Sam and assured them I was all right, I think. Buddy was excited and said that what had just happened between the table and me was "psychokinesis" or "PK"—the moving of objects by thought alone. It sounded like a lot of hocus-pocus nonsense, but there was no denying that the table *had* moved. So, now "moving things" had entered the picture—on top of the mysterious car clicks. Were the two events somehow connected? I didn't know what to think anymore. It was so unsettling, frightening yet exciting. I wanted it gone, but I also wanted it to go on. . . .

Wonder and curiosity prompted me to try to re-create the feelings that had overtaken me—and perhaps the effects—but this time voluntarily. I just hoped I wouldn't feel so sick again. Looking discreetly around the crowded restaurant, Buddy, Sam, and I selected as my target a heavy wooden table like ours at which six businessmen were seated. I began to concentrate intensely, vividly imagining that the table across the room was on my back. Almost immediately I began to breathe quickly, deeply. Then, in my mind, I tried to shake it off. After a minute of total focus, I saw that the table across the room was beginning to move. It was quivering so much that the men were shouting at one another, "Hey! Stop playing around! Quit shaking the table!" and were looking around, trying to find the joker. I marveled at the fact that this time I was much more aware of everything going on. I found I could hold on to my visualization and watch what was going on at the other table simultaneously.

The concentration it took for me to move the second table was a great strain but not quite as bad as before. I felt weak, but incredibly thrilled. Knowing that I had actually moved that table *with my mind* overshadowed any physical depletion.

My friends were speechless.

I tried to fix my sights on coming back to reality. Reality . . . What was real anymore? Buddy and Sam had seen the tables move, and that much was a great relief. But this couldn't really be happening! The whole thing was becoming too scary, and I felt as if I had entered an episode of the proverbial "Twilight Zone."

It was late winter of 1973. Clairvoyance (literally "clear sight")—the ability to perceive events beyond the range of the five senses—intruded into my increasingly confused world. Coming out of a movie theater in Greenwich Village with Buddy after seeing Mel Brooks's *The Twelve Chairs,* I suddenly "saw" a blue room and a fire in my mind. I had a strong feeling that Buddy should call his wife, who was at their condominium in Miami, Florida. When he did so about fifteen minutes later, he learned that there had been a fire in their living room—the firemen were just leaving! The room, of course, was decorated in shades of blue. Shirley kept asking Buddy how he knew, because she wasn't going to tell him. Buddy told her I had a vision of it at the time it happened.

We headed home, trying to remember funny parts of the movie to block out the stranger story. I was chilled to the bone when the now anticipated car clicks spelled out one of the most prophetic and perplexing messages: DEAN YOU WILL HAVE ALL POWERS USE THEM CAREFULLY.

This was happening a little too fast for me. I no longer felt like the captain of my own ship—there was someone else at the helm.

I had another odd vision soon after. I was driving on the Belt Parkway in Brooklyn, on my way home from a friend's house. The radio was broken and I was enjoying the silence, when I suddenly received a distinct mental picture of a fire burning on top of water. What *is* this with fires? Trying to shake this peculiar image, I opened the car window to get some fresh air, but the vision of fire on water remained strong and filled my head.

Preoccupied, I unintentionally drove past my exit on the parkway. I had reached Seagate, a private community at the tip of Brooklyn, when I heard shrill sirens and saw flashing lights as police cars sped down the usually quiet streets. Driving closer to the shore, I saw a glow on the water—a fire! I stopped a policeman, and he explained that two oil barges traveling in opposite directions had collided under the Verrazano-Narrows Bridge, which connects Brooklyn to Staten Island. A subsequent explosion had caused the oil spilling on the water to burst into flames. The police officer said help was needed in getting survivors out of the freezing water. As I hurried to the water's edge to join the chain of volunteers already there, a shiver ran down my spine. My eerie premonition had come true!

I entered the "human chain" that eased into the icy shoulder-deep ocean water, retrieving people who had endured the fiery collision. Afterward, a fireman put a heavy wool blanket around my shoulders and handed me a cup of steaming coffee. I sat down on the sand and stared out at the mayhem. I just couldn't believe I'd seen this picture in my mind forty-five minutes before!

The next day there was a picture and the headline "Fire and Water—Tanker Collision" on the front page of the New York *Daily News.*

At this point, I felt as though I were enduring the rigorous basic training of the nonexistent *Experiential Encyclopaedia of Paranormal Abilities from A to Z.* Over the next three- to four-week period, as Buddy and I and sometimes Sam drove to and from work, we were the first ones at the scenes of many car accidents. Instead of my former attitude of rubbernecking and waiting for the next guy to help, an unfamiliar affinity with humanity would overcome me, and I'd rush forward. Buddy was usually too paralyzed to move, suspended in that state of animation when you're involved in or watching an accident and everything goes in slow motion. Alone, I either pulled open a crushed or jammed door or kicked in a window of a burning car, drawing people out with strength that belied my size.

After I freed these various people from their mangled cars, to everyone's amazement, including mine, they never had a scratch on them. I remember so many times after these accidents, just sitting on the street curb or the side of some highway, overwhelmed with tears and emotion—happy tears that these people, aside from being shaken up, were not only alive, but completely unharmed.

The frequency of these vehicular encounters eventually tapered off, but I was already beginning to experience a more loving, benevolent caring for mankind that made me feel anatomically unusual and special.

But it sure took a lot of convincing on Buddy's part to get me to go with him to see some close friends of his who, a year earlier, had lost their seventeen-year-old son in a tragic auto accident. They were both deeply depressed and still grieving for their only child.

I said to Buddy, "What do you expect me to say to these people? I don't even know them. I'm not a grief counselor or a priest. What could *I* possibly say that would make any difference?"

All of a sudden, the door clicks started going crazy. The message read, YOU WILL KNOW.

As Buddy and I were let into the large house in Rockaway, I was filled with an eerie sensation. The couple were pleasant although morose, but it wasn't they who gave me the willies—it was something that I had never felt before, something less tangible. As soon as we sat down in the living room, an unexpected symphony of consoling words started pouring from my mouth, words I'd never used before. It was very startling—I felt like a puppet with some other "source" pulling my strings and controlling what I was saying. And these foreign words of mine really seemed to soothe the couple. It was pretty amazing.

But as these words of comfort spilled from me, I suddenly saw what looked like a large area of thousands of tiny, shimmering dots form a humanlike apparition standing next to the china hutch in their dining room. As I blinked and tried to refocus my eyes, these quivering dots of light took the form of a young man, about five feet ten inches, with a Buster Brown haircut, a large nose, and severe acne. I really could not believe what I saw. Without warning, the manifestation of lights glided through the living room and right past us, and then sprinted up the stairs!

I was stuttering, trying to tell these nice people what I'd just seen, when the mother interrupted me and yelled in joy, "I hear his footsteps going up the stairs! I know it's him!"

The woman jumped up, opened a drawer in the china hutch, and brought out a picture.

I was stunned. It was a photo of the deceased son, and it was absolutely identical to the specter I'd seen! So now, what was this? I didn't believe in ghosts . . . I did not! But I'd just seen one!

Buddy and I left shortly after and talked about my vision repeatedly.

About a week later, Buddy told me he'd gotten a phone call from these friends we'd visited, and an amazing change had come over them since we were there. For the first time since their son had been killed, they felt a sense of peace and closure about the tragedy and were going on a long vacation to plan the rest of their lives.

They'd thanked Buddy for bringing me over—somehow they felt a connection between me and their newfound acceptance.

I didn't know what to think, but I was certainly glad these lovely folks now had their lives back. I asked Buddy if they had sensed their son's presence again since we were there, and he said he had asked, but no, they had not. They believed their son was finally at rest.

The phenomenal car clicks continued over a fourteen-month period, and Buddy's Buick had become like an old friend. Buddy and I continued questioning each other for reality checks, to make sure we were actually experiencing what we were. It was all too hard to believe, but seeing is believing. A ritual was firmly in place: Most days, Sam met us at the store, and we all took a slow stroll to the parking lot, where our friend, the car, waited for us. There was still great anticipation and nervousness—we never knew what to expect each night. Many times we would go first to some restaurant and debate the questions we would ask on the way home. Somehow, once we were in the car's unusual atmosphere, many of the carefully formed questions flew from our minds.

What continued to be evident was that the clicks responded only when *I* was in the car. This had always made me uncomfortable. I mean, why not Buddy? It was *his* car! *He* was the one into reading about esoterica and studying the paranormal, not I. This was all new territory for me. And what about Sam? He was a kind, gentle soul . . .

Perhaps this whole damn thing was one big mistake. Maybe when this "source" sent down these "bulletins," they were meant for a different car—one with vicars or rabbis in it. . . . Maybe these communications were delivered to the wrong car! It sure kept me guessing.

I had less and less time to spend with my groups and musical aspirations. My new world was absorbing me, obsessing me. And Buddy was impossible, for he kept trying to see how we could benefit financially from our "friend" and the information we could get: "Hey, Dean, let's head over to Atlantic City—maybe we'll hit the jackpot . . . with a little help from our 'friend.' " What a provocateur. But this never hit my truth bell, and I knew intuitively that my new gifts were not to be used in this manner. I always refused.

By this time, we tried to ask only what we considered to be important questions, but sometimes Buddy's and Sam's queries reverted to their own personal lives, like if the business was going to be robust the next day—Buddy had a one-track mind. Sam would ask career-oriented ones, like if he was going to become the rock star he dreamed of (the answer was no). I usually felt it inappropriate to ask inane or personal questions. There were more serious things to find out.

"When is the Vietnam war going to end?"

We were given the precise, accurate date. The information was always astounding, and the predictions unerring.

But I was still human, and especially interested when Buddy asked about my ex-girlfriend and me. Buddy knew that Rochelle was still on my mind, and he knew also that I shied away from asking about myself, but if I *were* to ask just one thing, it would have been exactly that:

"Will Dean and Rochelle ever get back together?"

I remember holding my breath, waiting for the answer.

Click, click.

A-ha! A wrong prediction, for the first time. I knew Rochelle, too, had embarked on a new life and had recently married. After being out of touch for many months, she called to tell me she was going to do this, and I was devastated. Rochelle sounded so unsure of herself, as if saying to me, "Tell me not to do this, Dean." For a person with all these newfound paranormal gifts, sitting there and hearing this over the phone made me feel absolutely *powerless.* I wished her well, hung up, and bit my lip. It was probably foolhardy, but I still felt intuitively that we would end up together, and I *wanted* to believe it.

Sam never really seemed to be jealous, just happy to be a part of our expedition into the unknown, but Buddy's envy came into play—and I understood it. How would you feel if it were your car and someone else got all the supposed "gifts" and you got nothing? But what no one understood at the time was that all gifts are double-sided—they come with confusion, obligations, responsibilities, and lots of pressure.

So I was completely unprepared for the shock I received when, after fourteen months, our car escapades came to a sudden unforeseeable end. The last message we received stated: DEAN THERE WILL BE NO MORE TECH-

NICAL MEANS OF COMMUNICATION YOU WILL RECEIVE MESSAGES AND VISIONS IN YOUR OWN MIND DO NOT BE AFRAID.

What the . . . ? This was tantamount to a "Dear John" letter! How could we be abandoned like this? How could my "friend" abandon me?! Us! Why now? Just as I was beginning to float after being unceremoniously dumped into a vast paranormal ocean. How dare the clicks do this to us . . . to me!

I was angry, hurt, resentful, and very scared. Now I was to head out on my own, with no clue as to where or how or even why. But what frightened me most was this: How was I to recognize the difference between my *own* thoughts and the "special" messages and communications I was to receive in my mind? I was disconcerted and freaked out. Wouldn't you have been?

Many weeks went by, and there was absolute silence from the door locks. When Buddy's two-year leasing agreement came due, we had some very serious and intense discussions about whether or not to give the car back. Though I still felt deserted and unsure about what to do, I told Buddy he should do whatever he wanted, as it was still his car. There no longer seemed to be any reason to hold on to this unique vehicle that had so effectively changed us all. Buddy also was torn, but finally leased a new car.

Then I decided to do what I thought any normal person would do—got really pissed and started to show off. I'd restrained myself for so long, but now I no longer felt the weight of secrecy. It was over, or so I thought.

I was still hesitant, even more afraid than ever to tell my family about my new talents, which were now becoming very much a part of me even though the clicks had ended and the car was gone. But one evening, while watching my sister Lisa, then fourteen, playing with her crazy Ouija board with a few friends in the apartment, I was seized by the impulse to strut my stuff. Though I had "played" with my psychokinetic ability at times—levitating pencils and such with Buddy and Sam—I had been afraid to push it too far. I didn't really understand what I was dealing with.

Lisa and her friends watched in silence as I got into the now familiar deep state of concentration, visualizing the definitive connection between my hands and the Ouija indicator a foot away—they were "one." As my breathing came in deep, short bursts, I extended my arms and pointed my hands at the indicator. I saw a stream of light pouring from my hands and melding into the object, and when I moved my hands, the plastic piece, which was now an extension of my hands, followed them across the board, onto the table, and off the table to the floor. Two of Lisa's friends became frightened and ran out of the apartment, open-mouthed and bug-eyed. My sister and her remaining friend were dumb with amazement. I laughed out loud. This was great! I had never exercised my ego like this! I felt a little bit like Claude Raines in *The Invisible Man*—laughing hysterically when he first showed off his "power" of invisibility.

The time was right. I decided to tell them about some of my strange adventures. Perhaps because Lisa and her friend were young and open-minded, I felt that though they might not understand what they'd seen and all of what I told them—neither did I!—they would believe me. Lisa seemed to grasp some of the significance because she promptly gave my secret away the next day, telling our older sister, Roberta, what she'd seen and a few of the stories I'd recounted. When Roberta cornered me, I knew it was time to share my tale with everyone.

It was Sunday, January 24, 1974, when pandemonium exploded throughout my family. My parents demanded to hear the whole story, and for the third time I tried to describe the events of the previous year and explain the changes that had taken hold of my life. I was flabbergasted that Mom and Dad took it remarkably well, especially when they repeatedly saw me psychokinetically move hard candies out of a bowl on the living-room table.

It was like a circus, and I was in all three rings at one time. My niece, Maura, then six years old, shyly pointed out an orange fruit-filled candy lying at the bottom of a glass dish full of cellophane-wrapped sweets. Then I raised my hands toward the dish, some three feet away, and closed my eyes. I pictured a thin ray of light connecting my hands to the candy Maura had selected. As I started to hyperventilate, I began to see the candy as an extension of my body. There was no room for doubt—my concentration had to be perfect, or I had to start all over. When I raised my hands, the orange ball started wiggling slowly up from the bottom of the dish, displacing the other candies, then shot out of the bowl to a far corner of the room. I crumpled in a heap.

The side effects of PK were always a serious energy drain. When my parents saw spasms shake my body and pain cross my face as I collapsed from the continued exertion of my performance, the harm I might be doing to my health was their greatest concern. After getting my composure back within a few minutes, I tried to explain that everything that had happened had been for the good and that it was hard to believe any of this could hurt me. (As I told this to my folks, I knew I was full of it. How could I possibly know what this would do to me or how it would affect me? Each time I'd felt chest pains and thought I was having a heart attack, but how could I have told them this?)

A couple of hours later, everyone was still buzzing about what they had seen. I noticed that my brother-in-law, Harvey, was rubbing his temples and forehead, complaining that one of his migraines had come on. I would not have been surprised if it was my little demonstrations and that I had brought it on! He headed for the bathroom to get some painkillers, but I called him back. I wasn't sure why.

"Wait, don't take the pills yet, Harv. Sit here in this chair."

I felt driven to place my left hand about half an inch from the back of Harvey's neck and my right hand just over his forehead, barely touching him. My hands felt guided, and it was as if I were an observer. I closed my eyes, and an oddly familiar feeling came over me—a feeling of that "oneness." At first I couldn't place the sensation, and then I remembered the woman who'd been hit by the car in front of Buddy's. When I had stroked her forehead, I had experienced the exact same feeling! I shivered as I made the connection between the two events. Then I found myself relaxing, breathing deeply but slowly, and imagining a connection between Harvey and me. I noticed my concentration didn't seem to be quite as intense as when I did PK. I did not hyperventilate, and I felt strong, rather than depleted.

After about two minutes I stopped and looked at Harvey. He was blushing, but smiling. He started hitting his forehead with the palm of his hand in amazement.

"The pain is gone!" he said.

As he told Roberta what he felt, she exclaimed that it was the first time in ten years that Harvey hadn't had to take a painkiller for his migraine.

I was more stunned than anyone. What had I done?

My parents were especially dumbfounded that a person could really do these extraordinary things, to say nothing of the fact that it was their own son doing them! But now a lot of things were falling into place for them: This was why I spent so much time with Buddy and Sam; why it usually took us four hours to get home from work; why I seemed to be shrouding so much of my life in secrecy.

For me, it was an enormous relief to share my secret with them at last.

3

Healing—Starting *a* New Way *of* Life

THE IMPULSE TO LAY MY HANDS ON MY FATHER'S back in an attempt to relieve his debilitating pain was the culmination of a series of events that had plunged my life into chaos. These episodes were so bizarre that there were many times I truly questioned my sanity.

I cannot recall a day when I was growing up that my father's back didn't hurt him or make him cry out in pain as he turned in restless sleep. There were many nights I'd be up, wishing I could do something to help him. I did not know then that one day I would be given that opportunity.

His trouble had begun during World War II when he was stationed on active duty in the Philippine Islands. He fell while lifting heavy antiaircraft equipment, and ruptured a disc in his back. That injury went undiagnosed for three years before surgery was performed. Ankylosing spondolitis, with its severe back and neck pains, plagued Dad thereafter, and eventually he was diagnosed as having a rare form of another type of osteoarthritis called Marie-Strumpell disease.

My father was eventually robbed of his mobility. As he described it, every move sent searing pokers of pain through his body. It usually took him two hours in the morning to wash and dress, even with Mom's help. I remember when I was young it was difficult for him to get down on the floor and play with me. He would do it anyway, happily and lovingly, but slowly and awkwardly. He always tried to hide his pain, and never complained to Mom, my two sisters, or me.

In January of 1974, my father had only a touch of gray in his dark, thick, wavy hair, but otherwise he looked and moved like a man much older than his fifty-nine years. He was short and stocky, and during the late sixties his back became increasingly hunched because of growing calcium buildup along his spine. Although he had a closetful of assorted corsets and back braces, in time he found it difficult to walk, even with a cane.

The idea of laying my hands on my own father had occurred to me just the day before, when I had tried, for the first time consciously, to heal by laying my hands upon my brother-in-law's head and relieving him of the pain of his migraine.

Incredible though it was, I seemed to have acquired some very unusual powers—the ability to move objects with my mind, to see events at a distance, and now, it seemed, even to heal. My parents were still reeling from this extraordinary revelation, when I asked my father how he felt about my trying to use this yet-unexplained force to try to help him. He readily agreed.

"Let's do it!" he said enthusiastically.

My father was not a flighty man. If he hadn't seen me move those candies and other small objects without touching them, I'm sure he would have sent me to a psychiatrist for claiming to do so. But he knew me well enough to know that I was sincere, and he knew I'd never been interested in psychic events or played with magic. Dad had seen me do remarkable things, and since he had tried everything to get relief from his pain, including all the treatments offered by conventional medicine, as well as acupuncture, he was more than willing to be my guinea pig.

And Mom was great. She was the vibrant family cheerleader, always encouraging me. Right from the very beginning, she was optimistic, supportive, and hopeful that I might actually be able to help Dad in some way. I myself didn't know what to expect. I had helped a headache, but could I help Dad's back condition? Or was it only pain I could ease? I regarded my attempt as an experiment to satisfy my own curiosity. It would be wonderful if my father found some relief, but I felt no pressure to succeed. I had absolutely no fear of failure, for I wasn't attached to the idea that I might have a true healing gift.

I led my father into the den of our small apartment, and asked him to straddle a straight-backed chair. He took off his shirt, showed me his scars, pointed out the different areas of discomfort, and told me in some detail how his problem had developed, much as he might have explained it to a doctor. I was rather flattered that he was really taking this seriously! And the information he shared was very helpful, for I'd understood his illness only vaguely before. Now I had more of a visual image to work with. Somehow I felt this was important.

Then I stood behind Dad, closed my eyes, and began to breathe deeply and slowly. Gently, I put my palms next to his lower back, about half an inch from his skin, directly over the scars left by his operation.

I can still remember the sudden and tremendous feeling of warmth. . . . That feeling of "oneness" again nearly overwhelmed me to tears. I felt such an intense desire to help him, to give of myself to him. This was my first realization that healing is like loving. As soon as I placed my hands gently on his back, I noticed how unusually hot my hands were. They were vibrating, not visibly shaking, but internally quivering at an incredible rate. Dad told me he was feeling these very sensations and that they relaxed him, much like a hot bath. He seemed to melt into the chair.

I felt that same warm, tingling sensation running through my own body, just like when I worked with my brother-in-law. In my mind's movie screen, I saw some kind of pattern, like a figure eight on its side, with light going from one end to the other. Then I saw heat waves penetrating the skin on my father's back and surrounding, engulfing, and entering what I imagined to be inflamed muscles, displaced vertebrae, and sharp points of accumulated calcium deposits. I had no medical knowledge—my visualization grew from what many of us generally know of the human body and from what my father had described to me. I felt as if something were *guiding* me and my hands.

For perhaps twenty minutes I concentrated on releasing and focusing energy, and then somehow I knew that the experiment was complete. My heart was beating strongly, but I didn't feel that enormous drain that always accompanied me when doing psychokinesis. Within a minute or two, I was breathing normally and feeling a little light-headed. It was rather nice. I walked around the chair to face my father. He was smiling as he turned his body at different angles. He looked surprised, and I could see that he was impressed—I certainly was!

"I really felt something, Tiny!" Dad exclaimed over and over to Mom.

"It felt like electricity and heat coming from Dean's hands!" He said he could still feel it, along with a soothing warmth. He got up, walked around, twisted his neck, and nodded with excitement. The muscle spasms he'd awakened with that morning were gone. He was amazed—he felt no pain!

As for me, I wasn't sure whether or not to believe him when he said he felt better. Honestly, I thought he was just saying it to try to encourage me—until the next morning, when my mother told me that he hadn't cried out once during the night. He had awakened without his usual stiffness and pain, and even his attitude was better, more hopeful. I thought about the possibility that I had helped him with my hands. Though cautiously optimistic, I had no idea if this seeming improvement would last.

I worked with Dad as often as possible between his long hours at work and my own hectic schedule. It was over the next few weeks that we all began to believe that perhaps my father's relief was real and would maintain itself, and we finally gave ourselves up to the joy we'd been restraining. But even with Dad's increased mobility and comfort, his job still placed a great strain on his heart and back. So, at fifty-nine, my father retired.

This meant that I could work with him more often, and within the next few months, the results of my treatments were quite sensational. Dad was free from the dreadful pain. He began to hold his back straighter when he walked, and soon he discarded his cane altogether.

When I was growing up, my father's various jobs demanded so much of his time that we weren't able to be together very often. However, I had always felt his affection. He was an extremely loving parent, and family was most important to him. We both were very pleased with our new closeness.

A few months after I had first tried to help my father with the "laying on of hands," my folks went to their family doctor. Dad was scheduled for back and chest X rays. They came home with incredible news—the X rays showed that calcification along his spinal column, the source of his pain, had lessened significantly, and that his spine itself had actually and definitively straightened.

I couldn't believe it. I had to hear it for myself.

Within minutes I had the doctor on the phone and asked how he explained the sudden changes, but he offered no real explanation. Indeed, the doctor was baffled. The X rays showed dramatic improvement, and Dad not only was standing much straighter, but no longer complained of the pains that normally accompanied severe arthritis.

The important thing, as far as my father and the family were concerned, was that he felt better than he had in years. I was elated, but even after marveling over the news, I found it hard to believe that my father could have gotten such relief from *my hands.* I could not stop myself from peering down at them—normal-looking enough. It was thrilling to even think of the possibilities.

Later that day, my dad asked me to go fishing with him on the docks at Sheepshead Bay. I was stunned. We'd never shared this type of outing before—he had always been unable to fish because he couldn't lift his arms. He told me it was the first time for him in thirty years. I will never forget watching my father cast the fishing rod that day. Holding the pole up with his arm high above his head, he turned to look at me with a grin, tears welling up in his eyes. Struggling to convey his feelings, he said nothing, just tenderly kissed the back of my neck, a loving gesture he had bestowed on me whenever I'd had a haircut as a kid.

It was then and there that I began to accept what I had done. For the first time I considered the possibility of healing as a serious endeavor. Many doubts and many questions lingered, but my highly unusual pilgrimage into a new way of life had begun.

4

Early Healings

AFTER THE MIRACULOUS IMPROVEMENT IN MY FATHER'S health became apparent in March of 1974, word of my "vibrating hands" and their effects on Dad's illness and pain circulated quickly. Knowing that I had helped him and Harvey, relatives and friends soon began asking, sometimes begging, me to help them with their health problems.

I was struck by how willing some people were to try the laying on of hands to relieve their various conditions. I questioned those who approached me about their ailments, which included backaches, migraine headaches, arthritis, multiple sclerosis, paralysis, and cancer, and their doctors' diagnoses and treatments. It seemed to me that medical science had run out of answers for most of them. And though I still had no explanation for what was happening or why, after our sessions together, some of the backache sufferers were without pain, a cousin's depression was lifted, and an uncle's arthritic arm grew less stiff. I was now working with family, friends, and strangers in my folks' apartment, and began to make house calls.

As I was persuaded to do more and more healings, my basic technique evolved. Before I would begin, I would wash my hands and then automatically concentrate on quieting my mind, blanking out all thoughts and tension, and relaxing my body by taking a number of slow, deep breaths. My intuition led me to these relaxation techniques, but I have since learned that they are very similar to other meditative exercises used in such disciplines as transcendental meditation and pranayama yoga.

Having relaxed my mind and body, I usually spent some time with each person, talking about the case, and worked with the patient for anywhere from five to twenty minutes, during which, it seemed to me, my hands felt guided to certain areas. I felt a definitive connection with each person I worked on. Indeed, almost all the people I touched claimed to feel a pulsating energy, like electricity, passing into their bodies, very often accompanied by a sensation of warmth, well-being, relaxation, and sometimes even a pleasant light-headedness. They either relaxed so much they fell asleep, or became so energized they could hardly sit still. Many of them cried tears of release, perhaps because now they were also more *hopeful.* These side effects seemed to be experienced by almost everyone.

Somehow, having a mental picture of the person's problem area was very important to me. If a person had a tumor, I would "see" the fleshy mass. Then I would place my hands about half an inch above the skin over the affected area, at the same time vividly imagining the diseased growth beginning to dissolve and disintegrate. The more realistically I could visualize the troubled spot, the more satisfied I was with my interaction. I found an old anatomy book around the house and scoured it for basic information.

Positive word of mouth brought more and more people wanting to see me for treatment, and it quickly became difficult to continue working full-time at Buddy's, so I cut my hours to part-time, reluctant to let go entirely. By mid-1974, I finally realized I would have to make an important decision: I would have to choose between my old life of music, and this strange and breathtaking new path that had turned my life in an entirely unexpected direction. Finally, after seven years and not without some qualms, I left Buddy's Music to devote my time solely to healing, enabling me to see twice as many people. I seemed to have a new and unforeseen career.

By that time, some of the people who came to me for healing had begun to give me small financial contributions, which I accepted because I no longer had a "normal" job. My parents agreed to help me, as usual, so with my small savings I thought I would be able to maintain myself. The decision to give up a conventional means of making a living was made easier by the gratification I felt when people reported they felt better after my treatments, especially after their doctors had given up on them.

I continued to see my "patients," as I now referred to them, at their homes and in my parents' apartment, and Mom and Dad took the invasion of their home in stride. Their generous financial and unshakable emotional support during this transition never failed to fill me with gratitude. They helped me in every way they could—they bought me a beautiful wood desk, which was given a prime location in the living room; a plush, brown Naugahyde recliner for people to lie on; and they even put folding doors between the living room and the den to form a separate "waiting room."

Later I would move to more professional quarters, but there was a certain charm to my first "office." Anyone waiting to see me was ushered into the kitchen to be fed cake and coffee and to be lovingly pampered by my mother.

Les Draizen, a jewelry manufacturer in his mid-thirties, had arthritis in his right knee. Even though the cortisone injections had failed to relieve his pain and stiffness, his wife had to practically drag him to see me. He was kicking and screaming all the way. After questioning him further about his medical treatments, I started working on his knee. A few minutes into the session, I saw his face turn a deep shade of red. He started hitting his knee, standing up and sitting down, and exclaiming, "It's gone! The pain—it's gone!"

Les had come to me boisterous and angry, but he walked out purring like a kitten. I enjoyed working with skeptics and received great satisfaction when they improved. When Les left, I was prompted to make some notes about his condition and his response. Somehow I knew it would be important one day. I was naturally a pack rat and rarely threw anything away, so it was instinctive for me to begin to keep some records.

One of the most challenging cases of those early days was that of Pauline Sheinis, a sixty-seven-year-old Russian woman with a thick accent, who had been partially paralyzed from the neck down and totally paralyzed from the waist down for more than five years, due to complications from a severe spinal abnormality that had developed during one of five strokes. From the moment I first saw her sitting in her wheelchair, I knew I was going to try to help Pauline walk again. I guess I felt pretty sure of myself—after all, I was actually helping the majority of people I was seeing.

On the advice of my sister, Roberta, and her husband, Harvey, Pauline's son Marvin, a real estate agent, arranged to pick me up in Brooklyn one drizzly April afternoon and take me to see his mother in the Bronx. Pauline was suffering from constant headaches, which sometimes brought her close to passing out. She didn't believe in psychic healing, but after hearing about the relief I had given Harvey from his migraine, she had agreed to let Marvin bring me to treat her. It never bothered me when someone was a nonbeliever. I once had walked in those same shoes, and even today, I am still a very skeptical person.

When Pauline, in her wheelchair, greeted Marvin and me at the door, I immediately had a strong feeling that I should work on her spine and legs as well as her headaches. I'd never worked on paralysis before, but this seemed as good a time as any to experiment. Pauline had nothing to lose, for her doctors had told her she'd never walk again. I had learned early on *never* to make a promise or guarantee to improve someone's health. My intuitive knowledge, which was growing all the time, told me I couldn't possibly hurt her—the worst that could happen was that there would be no change in her already useless legs.

We sat for a while at the kitchen table, and Pauline talked. Her headaches had become so agonizing that it was sometimes difficult for her to think or even to breathe. At one point she had sought help at a special headache clinic, but the medication they had administered hadn't even taken the edge off her pain.

After making notes on Pauline's history (by now I was keeping documented accounts of all my healing sessions), I wheeled her into the living room. I stood behind her, closed my eyes, and felt myself slipping into a calm, healing state. When I touched her shoulders, she jumped and asked me if I had a vibrator under my skin. I laughed—I'd been asked this many times before—and showed her that I was using only my hands. Then I placed my hands in another position—one on her right temple, and the other on the back of her head. This combination of points felt right—another intuitive feeling that I was learning to listen to and trust. I focused on trying to balance her body's energies, to help catalyst or stimulate her own healing system. I sensed my energy flowing smoothly into Pauline's body, and moments later she quietly murmured that her headache was gone. She called to Marvin and her husband, Harry, that the pain in her head had vanished.

Then my hands were led first up and then down Pauline's spinal column, then to her hips, her ankles, and to points under her knees and arms. She surprised me when she asked if I was working on her paralysis. I explained that it was only an experiment and that she shouldn't expect anything to come from my attempts. Pauline assured me she was happy just to receive relief from her unrelenting headaches.

Because it was difficult for Pauline to travel in her wheelchair, I began visiting her twice a week, and soon I thought of her and Harry almost as grandparents. Whenever I stopped by, we'd sit and talk over the bagels and coffee she'd prepared for my arrival. After about a month of treatments, Pauline began to feel pain in her legs. Now this stopped me in my tracks! Pauline explained to me that to feel *any* sensation at all in her dead limbs was an unexpected and welcome miracle. Perhaps I was regenerating nerves? This was something to think about.

Within another three or four weeks, the discomfort diminished, but Pauline's overall sensation continued to grow. Soon she could flex her big toe, and then, slowly, she gained control of all her toes, her ankles, her knees. Finally she was able to work herself out of her wheelchair and onto crutches, for the first time in five years. After several months of sessions, Pauline was able to move quite well with two crutches, then two canes, and ultimately she was able to walk without any support at all.

It wasn't until January 2, 1975, that Pauline's recovery really sunk in. Trish Reilly at *CBS Evening News* in New York had gotten wind of my healing efforts and featured me on that evening's news. Pauline was my "star," with a generous supporting cast of other people I had helped. The film and sound crew crowded into the building and our small apartment. Curious neighbors were strewn all over the street in front of the apartment house and hanging out of their windows, watching Pauline make her way down the front steps slowly but surely on her crutches.

At six o'clock and again at eleven o'clock, I watched the tapes of her moving steadily on her crutches. I found myself shaking my head in wonder.

My God, I said to myself, *she got out of that wheelchair!* I felt lightheaded with accomplishment, and eminently proud.

•

Rabbi Israel Solomon was in his late forties, short and round, and very jovial, despite the fact that he was in great physical anguish. He had bone cancer, and the prognosis was poor—the cancer was in his ribs and spine. He'd been through chemotherapy and an enormous number of radiation treatments, but to no avail. He was dying. This was my first cancer case, and I was determined to have a positive effect.

Although I'm not religious, I believe in a "higher source." Rabbi Soloman was a warm man, encouraging me to think and talk. I opened up about myself more to him than to anyone else at that time. We explored some possible meanings behind my gifts and discussed different theories regarding my healing "mission." However, I felt the need to keep my approach scientific and medically oriented. But we had some great talks! He would tell me also that many times when he was in pain, he'd have only to think about me, and the pain would subside. He said that at those times, he could almost smell my aftershave. (It was probably Paco Rabanne at that time.) I always looked forward to seeing him.

After about six treatments in six weeks, the rabbi's health seemed to be improving. He returned to work with his congregation. Then, unexpectedly, he suffered a relapse. He called me from the hospital and asked me to come there to treat him. Of course I would! But as it turned out, his relatives wouldn't let me in, and there was a bit of a scene at the hospital. They were rigid, Orthodox, and narrow-minded people, and they just didn't believe in psychic healing. Their claim was that his illness and imminent passing was God's will, but I found that very difficult to accept. They forbade me from seeing him or even talking to him anymore. I felt terribly hurt and was very worried about this wonderful man. I felt helpless.

Shortly after I was rebuffed by Rabbi Solomon's family, I heard through another client that the rabbi had passed away. An emptiness consumed me. The loss was especially hurtful, for he had called for me and his relations had prevented it. I couldn't help but think that if I had been able to treat him just one more time, it might have made the difference, it might have helped. Rabbi Solomon was the first person I ever treated who died despite my attempts.

Back then, I was quite naïve about attitudes toward healing. Now I know that probably 90 percent of the people who come to see me for help will want to hide it from someone—relatives, friends, and especially immediate family. It's now easier for me to comprehend that people fear what they don't understand. Many people believe only in what they can see, hear, smell, touch, and feel—and I can certainly appreciate that attitude, considering what I've been through. Also, people don't like change, for change disrupts their routine, comfortable states. Usually, most relatives of ill people know only what their doctors tell them, and they accept the traditional Western medical ways, even though they comprehend very little about them either. They are closed off to any therapy they don't understand, and will object with great hostility to any possible "false" hope given to their sick loved ones.

Another interesting case that brought this point home and made me begin to question people's attitudes started simply enough with a phone call from the actor Al Pacino. He'd heard about my work through some colleagues and wanted me to see his good friend who was at Columbia Presbyterian Hospital in the Bronx. He had a rare form of lung cancer that had metastasized through both lungs and other organs, and was on oxygen. Al felt that his friend was terminal, but he didn't want to give up hope. Would I see his buddy that night?

Al made special arrangements with security at the hospital, and they let me in through a special entrance at one o'clock in the morning. As soon as I walked through the door, a strong antiseptic smell special only to hospitals made its assault and permeated my nose.

I was shocked when I saw how young and incapacitated this man was. He looked only a few years older than I—much too young to be dying from such a horrible disease. I just didn't realize that cancer struck regardless of age. How innocent can one be?

I was almost overwhelmed with the harsh odor of formaldehyde in the sterile intensive care room. It was very quiet except for the soft hiss the oxygen nose canula made, as this dark-haired man struggled to breathe. After a quick introduction to the kind person watching over him, I began to lay hands on Al's friend. Immediately, a sense of his gentleness consumed me. I did my best to pump this frail, dying man with as much "life force" as I could muster in order to try to "jump-start" his own healing mechanism.

For the moment, I had to put aside my profound questions about the fairness of life, and I continued to lay my hands around his head, neck, and lungs. Our interaction concluded, and Al and his friend were profuse in their appreciation that I was there, trying to help a stranger through a difficult period. It had gone very well, as far as I was concerned.

Perhaps it went *too* well. The following day, Al called me with a report: After I'd worked with his friend, he began to respond very favorably and was able to breathe better on his own, without the aid of the previously necessary oxygen. And he was more comfortable and animated than he'd been in months. Al was excited. However, I heard a "but" in his voice, and waited to hear the unimaginable—the parents didn't want me to see him again! They were very religious, strait-laced Catholics, and felt I was keeping their son alive by "unnatural means."

Three weeks later, Al's friend died. Al was very grateful for my attempt and felt that if I had continued my work with him, he might still be alive.

I couldn't believe it! How strange—a man improves from a horrible situation and the parents put a stop to it because of a lack of understanding and superstitious beliefs. I was beside myself with frustration and angrily questioned God, Allah, Jesus Christ, whoever, "Whose side are you on, anyway? What the hell is this all about?!" I received no answer. . . .

This was a poignant experience for me for other reasons. It was the first time I had disconcerting fears about whether or not cancer was contagious. It never crossed my mind when I had worked with Rabbi Solomon, but because Al's friend was so young, much nearer my own age, I related to it more. There had been a couple of times when, because I believed I had to feel someone's pain to better treat them, I had a sudden headache or felt excruciating pain that was identical to what my patient was experiencing. Gratefully, the pains were always gone by the end of the session, but somehow this was different and dangerous ground. I finally convinced myself I would not take on the cancer or any other illness, but also realized I'd better be much more careful about my need to *feel* anyone's problem. I knew if I was afraid of catching cancer just by being with someone who had it, then other people must feel that way too. What a terrible misconception!

The night I worked with Al's friend, I knew that I would not feel or take on anyone's negative symptoms or illnesses again. Mentally, I put up a defensive shield to protect my own energy and immune systems. It made a great difference in my confidence—I became less fearful about my own health. (You can do this, too, the next time you visit someone who is ill in the hospital or at home. Before walking into their environment, "see," erect, and completely surround yourself with an invisible, safeguarding shield or cocoon made of thick white healing light, and consciously say to yourself, "I *will not* catch or take on any imbalance or sickness. My own immune system will continue to keep me strong and healthy." It's simple, and it works!)

I realized I had a lot to learn about cancer and its frightening effects on people. This was the beginning of a lifelong battle—the "why" and "how" questions would fill my mind for years to come. I decided to begin to do everything possible to try to educate people, help dispel their fears, and promote the education of the potential positive benefits of the laying on of hands. I was then certain that I wanted to be involved with cancer research.

During these early months of my new healing career, I had been thrust into the center of my own emotional cyclone. The amount of success was almost overwhelming, but it became enormously satisfying for me to be able to bring smiles, tears, joy, and gratitude to the faces of people who had given up hope. Of course there were times when I failed, and it devastated me.

As I plunged deeper and more irrevocably into my new life as a healer, I saw less of Buddy and Sam than I would have liked, and sometimes missed the good old days in the car. I missed my groups and the exciting world I had given up. But it became essential for me to find out everything that might be known about my healing abilities. The same questions came back to me again and again: Why did *I* seem to have this special gift? Was I born with it? What *really* was happening when I concentrated on releasing "energy"? Why did most of the people I treated feel better immediately or within a relatively short time? And why didn't they *all* get better?

My search for answers had begun.

5

My Quest *for* Answers

MY FAMILY'S UNCONDITIONAL SUPPORT HELPED direct me in my search for information and guidance about my unconventional abilities. One of their inquiries led me to a social worker/psychologist at Nassau Community Hospital on Long Island, who was familiar with psychic phenomena and eager for me to contact him.

Naturally, I was hesitant, afraid the doctor might think I was some kind of nut, but the desire to learn more about healing and other psychic events pushed me to call. He listened intently to my story and then recommended that I contact Dr. Karlis Osis, then director of New York's American Society for Psychical Research (ASPR), at that time one of the main East Coast bodies devoted to research into parapsychology. He thought Dr. Osis might be able to provide some insight to my questions.

In the four-story brownstone on the Upper West Side of Manhattan that housed the American Society for Psychical Research, Dr. Osis, in his sixties, towered over me and spoke with a Slavic accent, while his youthful, curly-haired associate, physicist James Merriweather, tape-recorded my account of the clicking door locks in Buddy's car and many of my subsequent experiences of telekinesis, clairvoyance, and healing. The two men seemed to find my story fascinating, but to my disappointment, Dr. Osis told me that the ASPR was not equipped to test healing. The society was focused on studying the existence of "life after death." Still, Dr. Osis and James were very interested in my healing work. We arranged another meeting in which to plan specific healing experiments that the ASPR might eventually conduct, so I felt somewhat heartened.

I was about to leave the ASPR when the phone rang and a voice yelled for me to wait. I returned and found James on the phone with Yoko Ono, the wife of former Beatle John Lennon. James was a friend of Yoko's secretary, and by coincidence, Yoko was looking for a recommendation for a psychic healer.

James quickly told Yoko about me, explaining that we had just met and that he really knew nothing about me other than what I had told him. To my astonishment, Yoko said she got good feelings about me, so James handed me the phone and Yoko and I made plans to meet at her home the following day. Yoko lived in the Dakota in Manhattan, a dark and somber building adorned with ornate gargoyle sculptures that was used as a set in the filming of *Rosemary's Baby.*

One of Yoko's assistants led me into the grand ten-room apartment, and when Yoko Ono appeared, I was struck first by her very small stature and then her incredibly long black hair, which reached well down to her thighs. I thought she was much prettier in person than in any photo I'd seen.

She invited me into her large kitchen, where we sat in director's chairs sipping tea and talking about healing in general. Yoko was worldly and sophisticated and spoke in a clear way. When the conversation turned to her health, she told me she had been suffering from severe fatigue. We moved into the next room, which was dominated by a dining table and a unique sculpture encompassing a cube and a pair of jeans spread across the floor, both painted silver. Yoko sat in a chair, and I laid my hands on her shoulders. Then, after a moment, I placed my right hand on her forehead and my left behind her neck. My main focus was to "juice" her immune system and generally strengthen and boost her energy level.

Ten minutes passed, and Yoko said that she could feel intense energy moving into her and that she felt stronger and more full of life. Yoko and I sat and chatted for another hour, then set up a schedule of regular appointments covering the next few months.

During the first session, I had noticed a small, red rash on Yoko's forehead, but didn't think much of it. By the time I reached home, a similar rash had broken out on my face in exactly the same place! Oh, no, not again! I thought I had learned to prevent this from happening, but I supposed I'd let my guard down. Then the phone rang. It was Yoko, calling to report that *her* rash had suddenly disappeared!

After I hung up, I rushed into the bathroom and studied my reflection in the mirror, staring at the inflamed, irregular patch on my forehead. I was outraged and yelled aloud to the empty room, "I *said* I won't allow this! I will not take on someone else's symptoms anymore!"

By the time I left the bathroom a few minutes later, the mysterious breakout was gone, but the incident made me realize once again that I must be more conscious of protecting myself. That meant it was imperative, through concentration, that I keep my own "energy charge" so high, so positive during healings that I would be unable to receive any negativity in any form from the ill person. Since then, no similar incidents have occurred.

I learned a lot during my interaction with Yoko—she was the first person I ever heard speak in "spiritual" yet nonreligious terms. Though I had always felt reasonably comfortable about donations I received from clients, I listened to Yoko's reasoning.

"An unrewarded service disturbs a relationship," she explained with a smile. "One must graciously accept fair remuneration for a service, Dean," and she gently pressed a check into my hand. "When one gives and receives, a balance is maintained."

Throughout my career I've encountered people who think that a healer who accepts money is "unsaintly," that accepting payment somehow taints the healing, and that one can even "lose the gift" by charging for it. I think this is nonsense. I don't believe in exploiting suffering people, and I've always maintained a "sliding scale," frequently treating many people for free if they were indigent, but I do think an exchange of compensation is fair for an attempted healing. I believed that with every healing, the person receiving my ministrations walks away with a little "piece" of me. My preference, of course, would have been not to accept anything at all, but how do you live in this material world without income of some sort? As my folks had meager funds, especially since Dad's retirement, continuing to live off my parents was even more distasteful to me. The lovely handmade scarves and homebaked goodies were greatly appreciated, but they didn't pay the phone bill. Had I been born with a silver spoon in my mouth, I would never have accepted a fee for trying to help someone, but I had to survive.

One afternoon while working with Yoko, she warned me that John Lennon was on his way over and that he didn't believe she'd been helped physically—he thought it was strictly psychological. At the time I was feeling extremely vulnerable to any criticism, direct or indirect, so this made me immediately uncomfortable. I myself was still trying to ascertain if I helped people physically or psychologically. But I clung to the idea that it didn't matter *how* I helped my patients, as long as they felt better and showed improvement in their health and attitude.

John arrived with a couple friends, and, challenged by Lennon's obvious cynicism, I felt compelled to defend myself. I decided to counter John's attitude with a little demonstration of psychokinesis. Let him tell me *that* was psychological!

Just like my Mom, Yoko kept a dish filled to the brim with brightly wrapped candies, and I asked everyone to watch. I proceeded to make four different candies jump out of the see-through bowl and fly across the room in front of John, Yoko, fellow musician Harry Nilsson, and a reporter for *Rolling Stone* magazine, Lorraine Alterman. My audience was stunned!

I knew I'd made my point when John requested treatment for himself. At the Pierre Hotel, registered under the pseudonym "Dr. Winston," John wanted what I call a "general relaxation" treatment and for me to work on his eyes—he wanted to try to see better without his glasses. John also wanted to experience what Yoko had repeatedly extolled—the tranquillity and sense of well-being that she felt after our sessions together. Almost predictably, John described the feelings of light-headedness and euphoria, and claimed that after my treatment, he did see better without his glasses.

Now John had another problem—his electric guitar wasn't working. Jokingly, he asked, "Do you heal guitars, too, Dean?"

Casually, I asked for a screwdriver, opened up his BMW of guitars, a black Gibson Les Paul, took apart the wiring, and fixed the short that was causing the trouble. I'd done this dozens of times before at Buddy's Music. It now played perfectly, and John fell to the floor, laughing hysterically.

John and Yoko were enthusiastic about my unusual abilities and they felt they should be made public. They started the ball rolling by arranging my first major radio appearance on the Barry Farber talk show on New York's WOR-AM. It was spring 1974.

I was a bit nervous talking before such a large, unseen audience about my new life. Yoko had warned me that the longtime radio host was generally unsympathetic to the field of psychic healing, but she thought his show would be a good forum for me to share my story. During the broadcast, Barry Farber respected my stand that psychic healing was an *adjunct* to medical science. I made it clear that I wasn't trying to buck the medical profession, but wanted to supplement it with an alternative therapy when conventional methods failed. The phone lines were still jammed with incoming calls long after the show was over.

•

On an unusually warm and muggy evening for early spring, I received a distraught call referred by one of Yoko's assistants. It seemed a young woman and her boyfriend were having some type of strange episode in which something very weird was going on. The woman on the phone, Susan, spoke so fast and frantically I could barely understand her, but her plea for help was clear.

By now it was hard to resist a call for assistance of any kind. So I drove to a rundown, grafitti-covered warehouse in TriBeCa, downtown Manhattan. Hesitantly, I stepped into the corroded, unstable elevator, and it made its way tentatively to the top floor, groaning and shuddering the whole time. I realized how on edge I was. There was a pervasive feeling in the old building that I could describe only as "evil." I was almost sorry I'd agreed to come.

An attractive lady in her mid-twenties, with long, brown, wavy hair, opened the door. When I noticed her shaking and her eyes swollen and red, I forgot my own concerns.

"I can't thank you enough for coming over so quickly. I felt you were the last one I could turn to," Susan whispered. "My boyfriend, Loren, has not been himself lately. He's been getting these vague pains in his body, and the doctors can't find anything wrong. He says he's hearing these 'voices' in his head, telling him to do terrible, sinister things, but he wouldn't be specific with me—and, I swear, in the past few weeks, his face seems to have changed into a stranger's, with hard, grotesque features. . . ." She lowered her voice even more as she continued, "Please don't laugh. I know it sounds melodramatic, but he's like Dr. Jekyll and Mr. Hyde. And that's not all. Things in the loft mysteriously disappear and reappear in different areas, and I asked Loren if he moved them, and he swears he didn't. What's happening? I'm so scared! Am I losing my mind? Is he?" She desperately grabbed hold of my arm as if she'd never let go.

I was trying to absorb what she'd told me and felt goose bumps rise up my body. She finally let go of my numb arm and went to get Loren. I wanted out of there! Badly! Now! But as she walked back with Loren in tow, I pulled myself together and put aside my own fears to try to help with hers. I told her to stay in the front kitchen area of the long, narrow apartment, and took Loren with me to their bedroom area at the opposite end of the apartment.

Loren was a nice-looking mustachioed guy wearing blue jeans and a heavy plaid winter shirt. I thought his outfit unusual for such a warm evening, but there was a distinct change in the temperature in their bedroom. New York was having an early heat wave, but it felt frigid in there.

"Loren, can you shut the air conditioner—I'm freezing!"

"What air conditioner?" he countered. "We don't own one, but you're right. Susan and I have noticed a real chill in this part of the loft the past few weeks," he said in a Midwestern twang. I refused the sweater he offered.

This place was really creepy, and I felt as if I were in some really bad horror film, playing the part of the "paranoid intended victim," waiting for his inevitable fate to befall him.

Loren was relaxed as he continued telling me about the problems they'd been having, and they had been accurately described by Susan. Suddenly, he became very upset.

He said, "Dean, I hope you're going to believe me, because nobody else does. I feel as though I'm possessed. I don't feel like or even act like myself anymore, especially since we moved into this place. I believe there's some negative force here trying to absorb me! Susan and I have even noticed changes in the way I look, and some of my close friends have asked if I'm taking steroids or some body-changing drugs—and I'm not! I'm not doing anything and yet I'm feeling some kind of strong domination over my will power. . . . Do you think you can help me? Can you give me an exorcism?"

I faltered. I was in way over my head with this one.

"But, Loren, I've never done anything like that before. Maybe you should call a priest, or someone experienced in this sort of thing. I grant you, there's something peculiar going on, and I do pick up some pretty weird vibes in here, but . . ."

Before I could turn him down, Loren interjected: "We've already had eight psychics, three white witches, four mediums, two ministers, and even a Feng Shui advisor here, moving all our furniture around for the best vibrations. Nothing has worked. I'm pleading with you, Dean. Give it a shot." He told me that he'd even contemplated suicide over this, but then he said the magic words: "You are my only hope."

Those last five words were to become my theme song for the rest of my life. Though I was now aware of some of the paranormal abilities I had, there were always new situations that proved to me that I didn't know everything about my capabilities—or their limitations. So I had to try. In my mind I placed a big, thick shield of protective white light around myself, and hoped for the best.

Wanting to get this over with, and almost prove my inability to help in this case, I had Loren sit down on a mat on the floor in the middle of the bedroom. There were no ordinary chairs around, only about a dozen large colorful pillows spread about Bohemian style. As Loren got into a lotus position, I stood behind him and attempted to lay hands on his head.

But the moment I tried to touch him, I got a tremendous shock that sent me flying ten feet backward! It felt like a bomb had gone off and I'd gotten caught in its powerful blast of energy. *My* energy had been repelled by . . . something! Simultaneously, all the lights in the whole loft started flickering, and Loren gave out a sudden earsplitting scream! I lay stunned, my fall fortunately softened by some of those pillows.

This was impossible! And straight out of *The Exorcist.* Would he twist his head around in an impossible circle and spit green pea soup at me?

Susan saw the lights fluctuate, heard the commotion and Loren's howling, and ran down to the bedroom.

Loren was now quiet, his head lowered. He was in some sort of trance, sitting in the same lotus posture on the floor.

I was scared and exhausted but felt I couldn't abandon the two of them like this. Now I felt challenged by the unseen hostile "force" that filled the cold air.

When Loren lifted his head, he stared straight at me, but through me, as if not really seeing me. Yet there was a malevolence about the look that was definitely aimed at me. His pupils had a reddish glow about them. Maybe it was just the lighting creating this awful effect.

After assuring Susan that everything was under control (who was I kidding?), I took a few deep breaths and calmed myself. Very cautiously, I tried to place one hand on the middle of Loren's forehead and the other on the back of his head. This time there was no electric shock and I was able to make physical contact. But at that moment, Loren began to scream again, saying alternately, "Get away from me!" in a low-pitched growl, and the next moment switching back to his regular voice, pleading with me to help him.

I refused to give up. I felt as if my energy was being drained and sucked right from my body with a powerful vacuum. Suddenly I began to shudder, and Loren started shaking in synchrony. Then came a loud *CRASH* and we both collapsed onto the mat.

This is how Susan described it to the two of us. The lightbulb right above us on the ceiling had blown up, littering us and the floor with tiny shards. Slowly, Loren and I shook off the fragments of glass. I was groggy and out of it, but Loren looked good, different, much calmer. When he finally spoke, his voice was his own.

"Dean, you did it! I feel better—like a fifty-pound weight has been lifted from me. You saved me! I feel light, good . . . like myself!"

Susan started to cry, and she and Loren hugged and then included me in their circle. They continued thanking me as I gradually prepared to leave. I was unnerved but subdued as I made my way back down in the elevator from hell.

Honestly, I don't know if Loren really had been possessed by some malevolent force, or just believed he was—but what was the difference? I wasn't sure if I believed in evil spirits taking control over someone. But I had allowed my intense curiosity and my need to be of help to push me into a situation I didn't understand and never wanted to be involved with again.

Thank God—I walked away from another one! I remember thinking. *I'll stick to healing.* You live and you learn.

But I was also excited and couldn't wait to call James, the associate at the ASPR who had befriended me, to discuss this latest experience with him and seek further answers to some of these mysteriously disturbing situations that seemed to seek me out.

•

When one begins to study a new field, one quickly discovers the existence of an inner circle in that specialty. One encounters, again and again, the same few names—the people who are most acclaimed, most active, most influential or otherwise notable for their accomplishments. As I searched for an explanation for all the unusual things that were happening to me, I began to get together with some of the people most prominently connected with research into paranormal events.

James Merriweather was stunned by my eerie tale of Susan and Loren and could offer little in the way of explanation. However, we met several times to discuss the possibility of getting the American Society for Psychical Research interested in healing research. In May 1974, he invited me to an ASPR symposium in New York, which he thought would be a good opportunity for me to meet some of the other people connected with the society. And there were many.

A number of important people in parapsychology were to lecture at the symposium. Among them were Russell Targ, a laser physicist from the Stanford Research Institute in California, and Professor Bernard Grad, from McGill University in Canada, who is best known for a variety of healing experiments conducted with Colonel Oskar Estebany, a Russian healer. Professor Gertrude Schmeidler of City College of the City University of New York, who conducted experiments in psychokinesis with psychic Ingo Swann; Jeanne Houston, a researcher with the Mind-Science Foundation; and Dr. Stanley Krippner and former ASPR president Montague Ullman, both of the Dream Lab at Maimonides Hospital in Brooklyn, also spoke.

This was my first exposure to the world of psychic research. All day long, in the large auditorium, reports on experiments were presented by one monotoned scientist after another. Occasionally there was a witty speaker, but, to be honest, after a while the program became tedious. So James kept me busy outside, meeting people, and I found this environment more exciting. An intellectual atmosphere prevailed at the symposium, and for the most part the people in attendance seemed pretty levelheaded, not flaky.

James introduced me to Helen Kruger, who was in her late forties, thin, down to earth, and a freelance reporter for the *Village Voice.* Helen had written a number of articles about the paranormal and was completing a book called *Other Healers, Other Cures* (in which I was eventually included).

Then Helen and James introduced me to one of the main guest speakers, Larry LeShan, Ph.D., an authority on psychic healing. This was not the first time I'd heard this name. Yoko had told me about LeShan and put me on the phone with him to set up an appointment for us to meet. He'd squirmed his way out of that one. Now Helen and James believed it would be important for Dr. LeShan to observe me in action and were certain he would be able to begin to answer some of the questions that continued to plague me. They genuinely thought he would help guide me through the paranormal maze.

It was apparent that Helen had to pressure the man into a meeting. He kept saying he was too busy and tried to put it off, but Helen would have none of that.

"What's the matter, Larry? Too busy selling your books to check out some competition or maybe someone with a *real* healing ability?"

She had set the trap. He finally took the bait and acquiesced to a meeting, where he would observe while I did the laying on of hands for some of his own patients. Helen insisted on being present, and I felt better about it. It was an awkward situation, but I was pleased to have Helen as an ally.

I was looking forward to this encounter because up until then, I'd felt a bit isolated. Meeting "faith" healers with a religious basis for their work was interesting, but I'd yet to meet another healer like myself, interested in a scientific and medical understanding of the process.

My dad proudly accompanied me to the doctor's office in the city. He too was excited at the prospects of understanding what was happening to me. He and Mom constantly asked around if there were any labs, societies, or anything that might help explain my new life.

As we waited anxiously in the small, dank, and poorly lit room, there was no sign of Helen Kruger. Where was she? She should have been here by now. I'd spoken with her the day before, and she had confirmed that she would be there, assuring me that she wouldn't miss it for the world. As Dr. LeShan's assistant led us into another sad, dreary room, I noticed a sly smile on her face. I was beginning to feel uneasy. LeShan, in his mid-fifties with grayish-white hair, glasses, and wearing an old nubby black turtleneck sweater, sat arrogantly behind his desk.

"I'm sorry, but your father will have to stay in the waiting area," he dictated.

I asked when Helen would be joining us.

"Oh, she called. Something came up and she couldn't make it," he calmly replied.

As Dad was escorted back to the waiting area, a heavy cloud of doom and gloom washed over me. I couldn't help but feel that something unfriendly was unraveling, and a wave of wanting out flowed through me. But it was too late—one of the patients was brought in. He was a middle-aged man, balding, with a painful case of tennis elbow.

The doctor leaned back in his chair, clasped his hands across his untoned stomach, and stared at something obviously fascinating on the ceiling. I began to work with the pleasant patient, and after about ten minutes, he told the mute doctor how unusual my hands felt and that his elbow already felt better. After another few minutes, I felt complete with the session and LeShan abruptly dismissed the patient without a word. Well, I thought, the doctor would probably call him over the next few days and check on him, but his observation was odd—no questions of any kind? No notes? No nothing!

The next patient was an older woman, with short gray hair and large glasses, suffering with a sacroiliac problem and constant pain in her lower back. She asked if she should remove the steel back brace she wore preventatively, as she did when Dr. LeShan worked with her. But LeShan insisted she keep it on. We both were surprised. The brace did not intimidate me, and the session went well. She thanked me afterward, saying she felt pleasantly rested and that some of the pain had seemed to ease. Again she was ushered out before she could say another word, and again the doctor made no notations.

I was perplexed by his approach. Before I could ask or say anything, LeShan requested I work on his arthritic left knee. I placed my hands on his knee and I could feel the energy flowing smoothly, but I was still puzzled.

When I sat down, he blurted, "Well, I see no evidence of psychic healing here. Maybe you should go back to your old job and do this as a hobby on weekends." Then he sat back in his chair, smug and thoroughly obnoxious.

Now this really ticked me off. "Obviously you had your mind made up before we even started. You heard them yourself—they both liked the treatment and felt less pain right away! And it's also obvious that you have no plans of even speaking with them in a few days to see if they are still feeling better. This is total bullshit!" And I stomped out of the office, gesturing wildly as I told Dad exactly what had transpired.

Dad was as irate as I was, and without first knocking on the door, he walked right into the doctor's office.

"What right do you have to treat my boy like this! He has a true gift and you are supposed to be a teacher, a doctor, a practitioner of what you preach—what kind of observation was that? You ask no questions of these people? How could you make a statement like that without following up on them? How dare you!" Dad was sputtering and red in the face, and I tried to calm him.

LeShan sat placidly and would not make eye contact with either of us. Was he scared that I could be competition? I didn't want his patients—I already had more than enough of my own. I wanted direction and guidance! Suddenly it was all too clear that this had been a waste of time.

"Who died and left you boss?" demanded Dad, outraged. We both turned and stormed out. It was difficult to absorb the fact that this man actually had the impudence to try to prevent me from healing!

When we got home, I called Helen, ready to lay into her for abandoning me, but she was already steaming mad. She told me LeShan had called her as she was leaving to meet me, and told her *I* had canceled the meeting so not to bother! She didn't know I saw him, and as I recounted the experience, we both were very upset.

This was my introduction to the politics of parapsychology. I knew this probably wasn't going to be my only run-in with him.

Several days after the debacle, Helen called to ask if I could come to her apartment to treat a friend who had fallen by her swimming pool. The woman's doctor had told her that she had strained her back and that it would just take time for the pain to subside. I went to Helen's place and treated her, and right there, the pain disappeared.

After her friend left, Helen began asking me more about the experiences that had led me to healing. Then, abruptly, Helen walked over to a bookshelf and returned with a cumbersome set of keys on a round silver ring. She asked me if I'd ever tried to do psychometry. When I said I'd never heard of psychometry, she patiently explained that it was the ability to discern emotion or information from an inanimate object.

I took the keys, sat back in my chair, closed my eyes, and emptied my mind of outside thoughts. Unconsciously I began rubbing the keys with my fingers, and like a flash I saw an image of a plain, middle-aged woman! Suddenly my hand and then my entire arm began to shake convulsively. My head began to pound. It was a struggle to speak.

"Something's wrong," I gasped. "I don't feel well. . . . This woman's dead!"

"How old?" Helen asked excitedly.

"About forty-five," I told her. "I feel something tragic, some severe emotional distress."

I didn't like the feelings I was receiving. Afraid to hold the keys any longer, I dropped them to the floor. The pounding inside my head and the shaking of my arm began to subside.

Helen had been watching me intently, hanging on every word I said, and she was obviously taken aback. The keys belonged to a forty-five-year-old friend of hers, she told me. The friend had just died of a heart attack, which seemed to have been brought on by a series of deep personal crises!

I was saddened but also excited that I had been able to perceive these pieces of information, but I didn't care for the physical and emotional discomforts that seemed to accompany psychometry. The experience was unnerving.

"I've got to call Judy!" Helen exclaimed, and she immediately phoned Judith Skutch, whose Foundation for Parasensory Investigation conducted extensive research into parapsychology.

That very night we went to see Judy, who at that time lived with her stockbroker husband, Robert, in a huge apartment building on Manhattan's Upper West Side. The elevator delivered us to two gold-trimmed doors, the private entrance to an elegant multiroomed apartment. A number of other people were also there to see her.

When my turn came, Judy—short, attractive, slim, freckle-faced, and very youthful in her early forties—listened closely to the account of my unusual experiences. She had already heard from Helen about my healing of her friend and the psychometry experience, and at Judy's request I worked on several people on the spot and helped them with various ailments.

Judy was warm and sympathetic, and I liked her at once. The anxiety with which I had approached this meeting seemed unwarranted when she said that her foundation would help support my healing efforts and involve me in some research it sponsored. She suggested we put together a proposal for the work we felt was most important, and we quickly agreed that our first goal should be to see whether I controlled an energy that could be measured scientifically. Now we were talking!

As Judy and I came to know each other, she told me how she had become so deeply involved in psychic work. For some time, she had been fascinated with the inexplicable incidents of apparent clairvoyance and telepathy that she, like so many people, encountered in daily life. She always wondered about odd coincidences: How did it happen that the name of a person she hadn't seen in years would come to mind, only to be followed by a call, a letter, or news of that very person? (I'm sure you've had the same experience.) Many people are too busy or skeptical to pay attention to such occurrences. But it was several seemingly psychic experiences with her young daughter that had led her to become involved with the ASPR.

For ten years, Judy had been supporting and campaigning for research into paranormal phenomena through her own Foundation for Parasensory Investigation. In 1973 she had been one of the founding members of the Institute of Noetic Sciences; another founder was Apollo 14 astronaut Edgar D. Mitchell, who did telepathy experiments on the moon. The institute's primary interest was the scientific investigation of psychic phenomena, and the organization had collaborated with Judy's foundation on several experiments. Judy also had worked for the establishment of accredited college courses in the study of parapsychology, and in the early seventies, New York University established a full-credit course, which she taught.

I found her interest and attention encouraging and helpful, and I was happy to find a qualified guide through the labyrinth of the scientific paranormal bureaucracy.

We talked constantly about the importance of doing research to verify my special powers. I agreed with her priorities, for a medical/scientific explanation and authentication of what I was doing was still important to me.

As I was introduced to various people in parapsychology, I learned more about how my abilities were perceived. Most researchers were stunned that I could apparently turn my energy on and off at will. I was told that many healers usually don't have such control, and some can perform only in a favorable and supportive environment.

From the very beginning, Judy's belief in my powers was evidently strong. But it was an unscheduled demonstration of psychokinesis that finally unleashed the full strength of her enthusiasm on my behalf.

I was sitting with Judy in her living room. My insides were jumping with nervous excitement. All afternoon I'd felt the need to demonstrate PK for Judy. I wanted to impress her. Borrowing the pen she was making notes with, I decided to make it trail my hands across her shag carpet. I dropped the pen about two feet away and automatically began to hyperventilate. As I concentrated on forming the necessary mental connection, the pen began to move. In a flash Judy was down on the floor beside me, an experienced observer obviously checking for trickery.

As usual I passed out momentarily from the exertion, and I awoke to find Judy holding my wrist and checking my pulse. When I asked her what my pulse rate was, she said I wouldn't want to know, but I could tell my heart was racing. Judy herself was pale.

Within minutes Judy was on the phone, calling associates in California, planning a research trip for me. I listened in as the next chapter in my new career was being conceived. Judy and I shared the same hopes and aims for my work.

Now I had a sharper focus on where I was heading. But it was lonesome being on this adventure without a true companion. In July 1974, I got an unexpected yet long-awaited call from Rochelle. It seemed she had heard the Barry Farber radio show several weeks earlier and was blown away with the topics discussed and that I was the one discussing them! The show had piqued her curiosity, and she wanted to hear more about it directly from me. She justified her call by explaining that she'd made a big mistake and was leaving her brief marriage and going back home. Our desire to see each other again was mutual.

I went to see Rochelle at her parents' house. When she came to the door and I saw her once again, with her lustrous dark hair and her huge brown eyes, I felt all my old feelings come flooding back.

We brought each other up to date on our adventures and growth during the previous year. It was reassuring and heartwarming that Rochelle seemed to accept the changes in my life easily and without skepticism—just amazement and fascination. I gave her a sample of a healing treatment, and she gasped when she felt electrical vibrations in her toes while I was touching her temples. She was brought to tears.

From that first evening, Rochelle and I acknowledged and accepted that we belonged together. We resumed our relationship, which had begun when I was eighteen and she was fifteen. Within days, Rochelle left her executive-assistant job to help me in my work, taking over the structure and organization of the daily tasks I not only abhored but had no time for.

In Rochelle I have found my true partner. Her desire to be with me, help me, and share in my search for understanding has made my strange life more sane. With her loving, positive attitude, she has grounded my high-intensity, live-wire personality; calmed me; and helped me normalize my unconventional life and career. We agreed to live together, and for the first time, I no longer felt isolated on my journey.

6

Getting Established

I WANTED ROCHELLE TO BE INVOLVED IN EVERY ASpect of my life, work, and research, and took her to my next meeting with Judy. They seemed to have an instant rapport.

Judy had a big surprise for me. She announced excitedly that the arrangements for my first research trip were complete. On the seventh of November—only three months away—I was going to California for a week of scientific testing. Yes!

The phone rang, and while Judy ran to get it, Rochelle and I talked quietly in the kitchen.

"I wish I could come with you to California," Rochelle said wistfully, knowing that neither of us was in a position to pay for her airfare. But before I could get out a word, Judy ran into the kitchen and said excitedly, "Kid"—looking right at Rochelle—"how would you like to go to San Francisco with Dean?"

"You're a mind reader! I'd love to!" Rochelle cried, throwing her arms around Judy. We never would have asked for this. Judy's sensitivity touched us both deeply.

And Judy was no fool—she was banking that my test results in California would be better if I were as happy as possible. If that meant Rochelle accompanying me, then Rochelle would accompany me. We were overjoyed and could barely contain ourselves.

In the weeks that followed, Judy thrust me into a dizzy whirl of meetings aimed at creating interest in my work and opening influential minds. She also needed to raise funds for my upcoming research, so there were introductions to prominent and wealthy parapsychology sympathizers. Judy freely arranged gatherings with potential supporters, and I enjoyed the challenge of trying to widen people's attitudes to healing, even though the pace was sometimes tiring. With Judy's verbal persuasiveness and my demonstrable touch, we were a winning team.

One of the first notable people to whom Judy introduced me was John Tishman, the realtor/builder of the World Trade Center. I found him to be a very down-to-earth and amiable fellow who, after receiving a sample, became impressed with my healing ability.

One Saturday morning, I was awakened by a call from John requesting me to meet him at the LaGuardia Private Air Terminal in Queens. He had a friend who needed my help. I didn't know what to expect until I found myself strapped into the copilot's seat of a small twin-engine Beechcraft propeller plane. This was to be my first foray in a light aircraft, and I was excited about anything to do with flying, yet a bit apprehensive—its paper-thin aluminum frame seemed so fragile!

John was small, about my size, with thinning dark hair. He seemed very much in control and comfortable flying. It was breathtaking as John carefully maneuvered the plane between the Palisades on both sides of the Hudson River. We were on the way to Newburgh, New York, for me to treat John's friend Jack Shays, who was also a pilot and a flight instructor. It was Jack who had taught John how to fly. In fact, this was only the second time John had flown solo. Of course, you can imagine how comfortable that made me feel when he casually mentioned this at three thousand feet above the ground!

Jack Shays was more than six feet tall, balding, congenial but reserved, and enjoyed the pipe that usually hung from the side of his mouth. He suffered from angina pectoris, a painful and dangerous heart problem. Doctors had told him that the blood vessels around his heart were partially closed, prohibiting the free flow of blood. Although he was only in his early fifties, Jack could suffer a heart attack at any time. Consequently, his pilot's license had been revoked. As I treated Jack, he seemed more worried about his suspension from flying than his current health problem.

Over the next month I treated him four more times in my Brooklyn location. I focused my energy into his blocked heart arteries to "Roto-Rooter" them open. After each treatment, Jack would go to New York Hospital to have an electrocardiogram (EKG) taken, hoping that the machine would reveal a lessening of his arterial blockage. I thought this was a brilliant follow-up, for the feedback I received helped me to know if I was on the right track or not. But each time, the reading came back unchanged. After the fifth test, I was disheartened and told Jack I didn't think I could help him.

He brushed my remark aside.

"Hey, I'm not looking for a miracle," he said. "Why don't we try a few more sessions? Maybe some people need more treatments than others. I'm willing to keep trying if you are. I certainly have nothing to lose."

Of course, he was right. Why should I limit myself by expecting medically improbably results, especially after only five sessions? I guess I was a little spoiled because many people had been helped by fewer treatments, but that didn't mean everyone needed the same amount. People are like various-sized drinking glasses, and it takes a different amount of liquid to fill each one—not right or wrong, just individual.

After Jack's seventh visit, he did, after all, find a miracle. His EKG was suddenly and inexplicably normal, and it remained that way. His license was restored after the unanticipated healing of his angina—a condition that usually grows steadily worse—and soon Jack was flying again.

His thanks were heartfelt, but not nearly as gratifying as the lesson I was reminded of: *Never* put limits on yourself. As Richard Bach so perfectly stated in his book *Illusions,* "Argue for your limitations, and they are yours!"

Speaking of limitations, there were new physical ones involving my body as I began healing more often. Before being a healer, I always needed to eat three meals a day, fairly equally spaced apart, and I used to have an intense appetite. Now, during a healing day, I could not eat much, if at all. If I did, all my energy would go to digesting the food and I would feel tired and useless. After a day of healing it usually took a couple of hours for me to unwind before I could even think about consuming anything. I would end up having one large meal fairly late at night, which was probably hard on my system. My liquid intake skyrocketed—my body seemed to cry out constantly for water, and I found myself drinking many quarts while I worked and afterward.

I began to notice other little quirks, such as no longer being able to wear jewelry on my wrists or fingers. Since doing the laying on of hands, if I wore a ring or a thin bracelet, I would get intense pain right where the metal was—even my watch had to be plastic now. This pain could get severe at times and would continue for a couple of hours after I removed the jewelry.

I also noticed that all my senses became sharper. This change didn't surprise me too much because in order to do this type of work, your natural senses need to be enhanced. But every good thing has a flip side, a negative resonant. Now, because my hearing was oversensitive, I could no longer take the subway. The loud noise would deafen me and give me a pounding headache.

Fluorescent lights and other bright lighting were much too intense for my eyes and also contributed to many headaches. It wasn't any better for my senses of smell and taste, either. The worse odors and tastes usually were heightened, rather than the good ones. In the long run, these changes were not hard for me to adapt to, given all the pluses of doing healing work.

The patience and persistence that Jack Shays instilled in me were valuable when I treated lively, distinguished Irma Bacharach, mother of composer Burt Bacharach. Irma was suffering with osteoporosis, a demineralizing or loss of calcium from bones. This degenerative disease, which commonly affects petite women older than fifty, can eventually make bones so brittle that they break from simple bruises. Irma, in her seventies, had such swelling and pain in her hips, knees, ankles, and spine that she could barely walk, and then only very slowly with the aid of two canes. In fact, when she came to me she bought a mirror for us to hang near the front door of the new Manhattan office, for she was conscious of her appearance and liked to fix her hair after she arrived, but couldn't manage the fifteen-foot walk from the waiting room to the bathroom.

After several treatments, in which I concentrated on rebuilding new calcium into her fragile bones, there was only slight improvement in Irma's condition. I was surprised and disappointed to think that she might be one of the few people I would not be able to help. We both persisted. Then, after thirteen weeks of continued work together, Irma suddenly made great progress. She was elated when she phoned to tell me that she had just walked fifteen blocks! Then she began to forget her canes, and soon she was completely pain-free. Irma told me her doctor announced that she had gone into remission. Fifteen blocks! I cautioned her not to overdo it, but, like most people who find themselves unexpectedly well, she wanted to enjoy doing the things she'd missed out on.

The feedback I received from Irma's doctor made me want to know more about her disease, more about medicine in general. Somehow, I felt that my having this knowledge would be important to my patients. When I had the opportunity to meet Irma's doctor at a family celebration, he immediately cornered me, expressing how impressed he was with her healing.

When I asked him how he thought I was able to put Irma into remission, he said, "I know you did it, but I don't know how. But I'd like to refer some of my other patients to you."

I firmly believed in traditional Western medicine, even with its obvious limitations, but now I felt I would need to broaden my range of information and medical terminology to best communicate with the doctors. So, I bought some medical books to study. I attacked the books with the serious intent of gathering support from the medical community.

I scoured through reference books, such as the *Merck Manual,* in an effort to gain a progressive understanding of health problems and their appropriate courses of medical treatment. My new career was taken very seriously, and I approached this different aspect with even more intensity than I had with anything else. I did not take my responsibility to people lightly—life and death weighed heavily in the balance.

Many clients who were helped by my treatments widened my circle of medical contacts by telling their doctors about me. Sometimes they had to suffer their doctors' skeptical attitudes. I was eager to share my ideas with any doctors who would talk with me, with the aim of setting up research at their respective hospitals or clinics, since I still did not know the exact effects of my treatments on the human body.

Rochelle was now screening and scheduling my patients. She would tell me about a patient's ailment, and I would research it in my books. I studied the symptoms, causes, and procedures usually employed to help the problem. When I encountered the new patient, I made it a point to find out if he or she had exhausted all conventional medical channels I'd read about before coming to me. I didn't want them to use me as a substitute for traditional Western medicine. I found that the more clinical information I had about a person's condition, the better I was able to visualize the problem area and then focus on seeing it more clearly—a tumor smaller, an artery opening, or a slipped disc back in place.

Some psychics and healers practice psychic diagnosing, but I always want medical confirmation. I believe that the mind can create illness and can cure. Some people are so vulnerable that if a psychic told them they had certain illnesses, their minds might actually produce the conditions. There were times when I inadvertently picked-up on different problems than those described, or would get a feeling of what an undiagnosed problem actually was. In those situations, the only thing I would do was recommend that the patients get second opinions, and then make my own notes of my intuitive feelings. Quite often, a patient would return and tell me of a new diagnosis that confirmed what I'd already written on the record sheet.

Before long, doctors began to consult with me on difficult cases. One such physician, Dr. Abraham Weinberg, heard of me from Judy and requested my help with a tough case of herpes zoster, or shingles. For two months, the patient had been suffering excruciating pain from swollen sores on her torso.

Working with the doctor in attendance, I concentrated on radiating energy over the patient's afflicted area, and I visualized a stimulated blood flow in the woman's body to help speed the healing.

Dr. Weinberg called the next day to tell me that the woman's pain was virtually gone and her sores were already less inflamed. I treated her three more times, and within two weeks the shingles disappeared. Dr. Weinberg said there was no medical explanation for such rapid improvement. At least he didn't say "spontaneous remission," which was the frequent explanation for my clients' mysterious recoveries. Of course, I surmised that the number of "spontaneous remissions" I'd affected already had *itself* become extraordinary.

At this time, Dr. Weinberg introduced me to Maria Cooper Janis, the daughter of screen legend Gary Cooper and his wife, "Rocky." Maria's husband, famed classical pianist Byron Janis, suffered from severe arthritis that was especially painful in his hands. It had a crushing effect on his career, and when I first met him, he hadn't gone on tour for a number of years. He was an intense and solemn man, but enjoyed my enthusiasm and found it contagious. He quickly responded in our sessions together.

I remember treating him backstage at an auditorium at Yale University, prior to his comeback concert. It was a memorable moment as Rochelle and I heard the beautiful and emotional strains of "Rachmaninoff" resonating to the large, appreciative crowd. As I saw Byron raise his hands and arms in a high and rhythmic wave with full control, I looked down at my own hands.

As quickly as Byron's fluid hands had moved across the piano keyboard, word of his surprising improvement spread through the music circles. I was contacted by another artist whose career was endangered, Leonard Rose, a virtuoso cellist, formerly a member of the New York Philharmonic, and part of the acclaimed Istomin-Stern-Rose Trio. Then fifty-eight and a handsome man, Rose faced a grave problem: He had developed a severe weakness in his left hand, caused by a pinched nerve in the back of his neck. In addition, he had tennis elbow—in this case, cellist's elbow, really—and the muscles in his arm were beginning to atrophy. Pain and weakness made it almost impossible for him to perform, and the threat to his vocation had left his morale at a low ebb.

During the five weeks of treatment, I would place one hand on the left side of his neck, and the other on his forearm. I would focus on the image of the calcium spur that was pinching the nerve in his neck getting smaller and smaller until it dissolved. Leonard improved steadily, and soon after, he left on a long-awaited worldwide concert tour. When he returned he called to thank me and let me know that he had experienced no problems with his arm and was playing his cello full-time.

Some of my patients themselves were involved with the world of traditional Western medicine. Kyp Susser and her husband at that time, Dr. Murray Susser, who was a member of the board of directors of the International Academy of Preventive Medicine, came to see me about a painful knee ailment that had tortured Kyp for five years. Dr. Susser and other physicians who examined Kyp's knee had been unable to find the cause of her suffering and restricted movement.

As I laid my hands successively on her forehead, her shoulders, and her bad knee, I visualized the overgrowth of scar tissue in her knee dissolving.

"It feels like an electric shock is going through me!" Kyp said excitedly. Murray, who was holding her hand while I worked, said he even felt the vibrations passing from her hand into his. That very night, Kyp Susser recovered full pain-free movement of her knee. I never had to work with her again.

Another patient was Dr. Howard White, then a clinical psychologist who had worked at the Kingsbridge Veterans Administration Hospital in the Bronx for ten years. He was a former dancer with the American Ballet Theatre. Howard had suffered a variety of unpleasant symptoms—back and leg pains, loss of bladder control, spasticity in his legs, vertigo, and other neurological problems—for several years, during which he had run the medical gamut trying to have his ailment diagnosed. To his chagrin and dismay, the doctors had told him his problem was all in his mind. By now, to my frustration, I was beginning to hear "It's all in your mind" a little too often.

The entire condition was a result of being injured by an exercise prescribed for him by a physician. His other doctors finally realized Howard's partial paralysis was not psychosomatic. In fact, he had severe spinal cord compression. Two protruding thoracic discs were pressing against the spinal cord, creating the paralysis and other symptoms. Emergency surgery, in which a couple of degenerated discs were removed, alleviated the pressure on his spine. But Howard was left with a great deal of spasticity, muscle atrophy in his legs, back pain, and deep depression.

Each time I treated Howard, I directed the healing energy into the area of his back where he experienced the greatest pain. I visualized a knotted muscle, sent the energy radiating into it, then "saw" the muscle become looser, more fluid. Howard responded quickly to our sessions. Within weeks, his balance improved, the spasms decreased, and, with increased movement, his muscle tone began to return. He was able to go back to dancing. By his own subjective assessment, his pain had diminished by eighty percent.

Before long, my office looked like a dance studio. A professional ballet dancer with the Canadian Ballet, Jeffrey Baker, traveled from Ontario for treatment. He was totally debilitated by colitis, an intestinal problem causing continuous diarrhea and severe abdominal cramping. He had lost twenty-five pounds in two months, and although he was under a doctor's care, his medication wasn't working and the pounds were continuing to drop from his already thin body. To compound his dismay, the prolonged physical trauma of his career had left his knees constantly sore, making it difficult for him to dance. He was terribly depressed.

Since colitis is believed to be a stress-related problem, I focused a large part of my treatments on calming Jeffrey's body. After the first session, he let me know that he felt much stronger. By the third session he was bouncing in. He had gained seven pounds in six days, the gnawing cramps he'd felt for two months had subsided, and his knees were less sore. In another two days, Jeffrey gained a total of almost ten pounds, and the cramps, the debilitating diarrhea, and the knee soreness all were completely gone. In a relatively short time, Jeffrey returned to dancing.

Then ballerina Merryl Ashley, with the New York City Ballet, came to see me with the ubiquitous knee problems that plague professional dancers. I held both of my hands slightly apart and three inches above her knee while I visualized the fluids draining out of the swollen area. I started to feel a tingling in my hands, and just as I felt this, she mentioned a tingling in her knee and a lessening of pain. Within a few sessions, she was back in form and dancing with greater ease.

My healing practice was beginning to fill me with a new wonderful sense of usefulness and purpose. After all, how can you compare being a musician with being a healer? Healing was far more important and gave me much more satisfaction than even demonstrating my unusual ability to move matter with my mind.

Lately, however, PK seemed to be harder and more burdensome on my body—it drained me even more than it ever had, and I took longer to recover. I noticed also that the more involved I was in treating increasing amounts of ill people, the more laborious it became to do psychokinesis.

For some time now I'd been concerned about the wisdom of my continuing to do PK. I felt I might be incurring permanent damage to my body, so before leaving for my California research trip, I finally consulted with a medical doctor who had a genuine interest in parapsychology. After a lengthy discussion with Dr. Steve Gross, whom I met through the slowly increasing number of medical doctors that were interested in my work, I was even more troubled.

He firmly told me that psychokinesis could very well be adversely affecting my heart, and stated the case of a woman, Nina Kalugina, who was famous in Russia for doing psychokinesis. She was documented as having various heart problems and possible heart damage due to the unusual stress of this little understood phenomena. I was strongly advised to stop doing blatant psychokinesis.

It was only then that I finally realized that PK was just another stepping-stone to help validate to me that I truly had a healing gift.

My thoughts always drifted back to the same basic, troubling questions: What was the "energy" with which I helped people? How did I assist these people? Was it psychological suggestion, or was I actually affecting the body clinically? Perhaps it was both. I began putting a lot of thought into my pending research and continuing my efforts to get answers in a field of study that seemed more nebulous than I had ever imagined.

7

My First Scientific Exploration

Founded in 1946, Stanford Research Institute is a problem-solving organization—a think tank—situated on a seventy-acre expanse in Menlo Park, California, just south of San Francisco and within a few miles of Stanford University, with which it once was affiliated. SRI has branch offices and labs in Europe and the Far East, and often works with federal, state, and city governments in the areas of health, education, and public welfare.

It was finally November 7, 1974, and Rochelle and I had just arrived from San Francisco airport. After dropping our bags at our hotel in Burlingame, we hurried over to join Judy at a smorgasbord luncheon. Also in attendance would be Russell Targ and Dr. Harold Puthoff, the laser physicists I'd met at the parapsychology symposium; parapsychologist Brendan O'Regan (a former associate of Buckminster Fuller) of the Institute of Noetic Sciences; and Dr. Ted Bastin, a quantum physicist from Cambridge University and part-time research consultant for SRI and Noetics.

I barely touched my food. I couldn't wait to tour the parapsychology labs. I was somewhat surprised to see that they consisted of two closet-sized rooms. I didn't yet understand the problems faced by scientists seriously interested in exploring paranormal phenomena. I was told by Hal Puthoff that most of the research directors at SRI looked down on parapsychology investigations. It appeared that only a few innovative individuals took on work in this controversial field, and they tried to work quietly, without drawing public attention to their activities. Puthoff and Targ faced a constant battle to acquire even the most meager facilities. The majority of funds for psychic research at SRI came primarily from private individuals, corporations, and parapsychology groups, while most other projects were government-funded and received substantially more money.

That first evening, Rochelle and I were in Judy's suite at the Hyatt Burlingame. We were joined by Dr. Ted Bastin, the intense and scholarly red-haired physicist; and by elflike Brendan O'Regan, one of the directors at Noetics. As we sat in the spacious living room having drinks, we began to discuss some of the forthcoming research.

I finally had the opportunity to pick some very intellectual brains, and the theories were flying. Actually, I didn't understand quantum physics or a lot of what Dr. Bastin or Brendan were saying regarding my energy—it all sounded so obscure—but I did get a sense that they too were on a new road of discovery. They hoped that I would be the one to help them further develop their ideas on how biological healing was stimulated.

I would have liked some quick, brief answers to my questioning, but there just weren't any. It seemed healing research was quite young, and they were hoping the results of my upcoming tests would help move them along on the path toward more information on this illusive energy.

I was delighted to oblige Dr. Bastin, who had a stretched ligament in his shoulders, when asked if I worked on sore joints. My energy was flowing with unusual strength as I lightly placed my hands on the doctor's shoulders. After a few minutes of directing my energy into his damaged shoulder and envisioning waves of healing force entering his inflammed tissues, I felt him relaxing under my hands. Bastin said he felt a tingling sensation and a soothing effect. The pain disappeared entirely.

He, Brendan, and Judy started discussing his reaction to my attempts, while I thought about doing a demonstration of psychokinesis. I had a quick flash of Dr. Gross's warnings, but I brushed them aside. If I couldn't do it for the scientists, doctors, and professional observers, then what was the point? These were the people who could make a difference in the comprehension of my abilities. Once again, I felt it was an acceptable risk.

I expressed my desire to do PK and asked Ted Bastin to drop one of the ballpoint pens in his shirt pocket onto the lushly carpeted floor. Rochelle and Judy immediately knew what I was going to do, and they cleared space in the center of the living room, moving the large wood table to the side of the room. Everyone gathered around me in a circle on the floor, on hands and knees, and watched in fascination.

No longer aware of my surroundings, I felt myself begin to hyperventilate. I saw a line of light connecting my hands to the pen, absolutely certain that if my hands moved, so would the pen. My breathing came heavier, and the pounding in my head was already an ache. Then I started to lean back, and the pen slowly started inching toward me.

Judy, Dr. Bastin, and Brendan were running their hands across the rug in between my hands and the pen, checking for chicanery, and they were stupefied by my performance. I backed up as far as I could, and then, as usual, I collapsed in an inelegant heap, thoroughly wiped out. Rochelle rushed to my side with a glass of water.

Though extremely drained, I was still pleased with my successful presentation before a group of highly trained scientific paranormal observers. I felt as if a weight had fallen from my shoulders, and as the two men lifted me from the floor and helped me onto the couch, everyone simultaneously expressed their different views on how I was able to do PK.

Rochelle looked concerned—she hated my doing this because of its effects on me; Judy looked like the cat who had swallowed the canary;

Brendan didn't know what to say; and Dr. Bastin went to a different end of the living room, sat in a corner facing the wall, and repeated over and over, "It's not in the books. It's just not in the books." It was a promising beginning.

The next day was set aside for relaxing, so Rochelle and I rented a car and drove from Burlingame to San Francisco's Fisherman's Wharf—a seaport area crowded with restaurants, the Ghiradelli chocolate factory, and tons of shopping. The view of Alcatraz, sitting isolated off the Pacific Coast, was sobering, but this miniholiday was a nice reprieve.

We ate a delicious lobster lunch and then had drinks on the pier. Rochelle and I had been living together at her parents' home for more than three months and, in a way, we felt like this trip was an early honeymoon—our wedding was planned for the following December, just a little more than a year away—and we used the unexpected free time to deliberate some of the details. But I must admit, I probably wasn't great company. I was in a beautiful city with the woman I'd loved for more than six years, yet my thoughts and our conversation kept drifting back to my forthcoming scientific testing.

Rochelle was still adjusting to our new life, in which she fully supported and understood my goals. She knew that though my course in life had changed drastically, I was basically the same person, striving to be the best at whatever I undertook. My intensity can be overwhelming to some people, and I was always appreciative that she knew me from the "old" days and accepted the magnitude of my passions. Our day in San Francisco was a leisurely repose to what I knew would be a stressful week.

The following day, rested and eager to begin work, Rochelle and I were escorted to SRI by Ted Bastin, whose shoulder pain was completely gone; Brendan O'Regan; Judy; and Dr. Jerry Jampolsky, a famed child psychiatrist who had published papers and books on child behavior in relation to ESP. We had a brief preliminary meeting in the conference room, one of the two tiny rooms used for psychic research, where I was given more details of the objectives of the first test.

Then Targ and Puthoff showed me into the next cubicle, where, on a narrow table opposite the door, they had set up a pendulum apparatus covered by a clear glass bell jar to block out wind and air currents. The twelve-foot-square room was crowded with equipment, various chart recorders, and an enormous wall-to-wall computer. Rochelle sat, quietly observing, and it was quite a tight squeeze in there.

The goal of our first experiment was to see if the pendulum, which was swinging gently in a steady computerized rhythm, would be affected by healing energy generated in the same room. Hal Puthoff would act as a patient, and I would lay hands on him, as well as indirectly try to alter the motion of the pendulum.

I didn't give myself time to think about whether I could do it. The outcome of the test was important, my confidence high, and the fact that I had displayed my psychokinetic ability two nights before gave me an added boost.

Hal settled himself in a metal straight-backed chair, and I stood behind him, automatically placing my hands on his shoulders. Because he had no specific illness for me to visualize, I absently began to send general energy into Hal's body, but holding in my mind a picture of the pendulum apparatus. With my mind's eye, I saw the pendulum begin to swing in a wider arc under the glass jar.

Immediately, Russell Targ, tall and lanky, with bushy hair, who was carefully monitoring the chart recorder, yelled, "It's moving! Hal, come here and look at this!"

"Russ, I'm being treated—I can't move!" Hal objected. Laughter broke the tension in the room.

After a few minutes, I withdrew my hands from Hal, blanked my mental connection with the apparatus, and the swinging pendulum promptly slowed and returned to its originally set rhythm.

When Hal got up and looked at the computer and instruments, he seemed genuinely surprised. He said he and Russell had never seen such dramatic and unmistakable change in movement before. When Judy rejoined us, beaming with pride, Hal excitedly told her that the initial results definitely warranted further testing.

This test marked the first time I had performed PK and a healing simultaneously. It was not remarkable to me, however, for I had always felt that they were linked to the same force.

I was exhilarated but also felt very depleted from it all. As Rochelle and I were leaving the lab, Hal told me we would attempt the same experiment the following day. It was understandable that he had to be sure that my conspicuous effect on the equipment was consistent and not an anomaly.

The next day was Sunday, and the lab was deserted but for our small group. During the second pendulum experiment, Dr. Bastin was the recipient of my energy. There was great anticipation in the room. Again, I felt very sure of myself, and I decided to show these men the real extent of my powers. Leaving one hand on Dr. Bastin's shoulder, I pointed the other one directly toward the pendulum several feet away. All of a sudden, the pendulum started to make longer, faster swings, tracing a wider and wider arc and finally sweeping so violently that it fell off its treadle!

Russell and Hal stared at each other and at the charts with controlled bewilderment. Finally their reserve cracked, and they yelled with delight, laughing, and shaking their heads in disbelief. I was very pleased to have proven that the previous day's test results were not a fluke, but I was beginning to feel queasy. I excused myself and ran to the men's room to vomit.

When I tottered back, my pallor was evident to Rochelle, and she encouraged me to stop for the day. I was really feeling awful but still waited around for another hour, hoping to feel better. Finally, I had to acquiesce to Rochelle's advice to call it a day. I continued to feel nauseated and drained, and figured that this could be an adverse result from the experiment with the pendulum.

Even though I knew everyone was disappointed with the day's being cut short, they were not nearly as disappointed as I was. Rochelle and I returned to our hotel, where she kept me resting in bed the remainder of the day. As I lay there, I started to think, *Is this how it's going to be? Am*

I going to get nauseous and feel ill after each attempt at trying to demonstrate my abilities? Is this what I have to look forward to?

I awoke early the next morning feeling fully restored. In the afternoon, Judy took Rochelle and me to the Institute of Noetic Sciences in Palo Alto, where we briefly met former astronaut Edgar Mitchell, who took us on a tour of the facilities. Then we crossed the Golden Gate Bridge on to Tiburon, a lovely little town across the San Francisco Bay, for an evening session with Jerry Jampolsky, the psychiatrist. Jerry had a combination houseboat/office overlooking the bay, and you could see the ferry passing close by his large picture windows.

Judy had arranged for Dr. Jampolsky, a handsome man in his early forties and casually dressed, to set up and supervise the monitoring of my brain waves, heart waves, and blood pressure while I treated John Peterson, a friend of Jerry's and a reporter for the *National Observer,* a conservative Washington-based newspaper.

John had been struck by severe back pains and had spent the previous ten days either lying flat in bed or crawling around his house. On top of that, he had a cyst on his knee. He was going to write an article about my efforts to help him.

I chatted with John, a personable, hefty guy with a full, dark beard, while Dr. Jampolsky began the long messy procedure of attaching cables for an electrocardiogram (EKG), which monitors heart activity, and an electroencephalogram (EEG), which records brain waves, to my head and chest.

Initially, John was slightly apprehensive, and we found ourselves nervously grinning at each other. But as we began to talk, he grew increasingly animated. He told me that there never had been a serious scientific study of healers, a fact he discovered a few months earlier when he'd requested a search for such studies in the computer bank at the National Library of Medicine in Bethesda, Maryland. I was surprised to hear that.

Then, finally, Jerry told me to begin the healing. I could tell that for the first few minutes, John's heart was beating at a crazy rate and he was unable to relax. Then I placed my hands on his shoulders, breathing deeply and steadily, and began to generate energy into his back. I focused on trying to ease the burning, stabbing pain. John said he felt my hands vibrating lightly. Then I tried to work awhile on John's benign knee growth, but the wires were distracting and limited my movement to this area.

By the time I felt the session was complete, John was in a deep state of relaxation. He reported that for the next few minutes he continued to feel strange vibrations moving through his arms and legs and said it felt eerie, somewhat similar to the nervous and muscular reaction that follows a supreme physical effort.

The day after my session with Dr. Jampolsky and John, Judy, Rochelle, and I traveled to SRI's biomedical division, where I was introduced to Dr. Erik Peper, whose specialty is the different regions of the brain. Dr. Peper wanted to use an EEG to look for any difference between the function of my brain and that of people who don't evidence any healing ability.

Tall, thin, and professionally attired, Dr. Peper had an extensive experimental setup in his labs at SRI. Before the test began, he attached long, narrow cables to several parts of my head. Once again I was covered everywhere with the sticky, white adhesive paste used to connect the cables. Then I remained in the small lead-shielded room, while he went out to a connecting room to monitor his equipment. Through an intercom, Dr. Peper told me, successively, to relax, to tense my body and face, and to speak, while he recorded average, or baseline, readings. Then he instructed me to enter my healing state and asked me to tell him when I felt I reached peak concentration.

Dr. Peper quickly determined that I had full knowledge and control of when I was in a healing state. A couple of hours later, when we were finished, he also said that my brain waves were "unusual"—whatever that meant—but that he needed more tests in order to define their significance. When Judy rejoined us, she promised to arrange further experiments.

On Wednesday morning, Rochelle, Judy, and I went to the Stanford University campus to meet Dr. William Tiller, an innovator of research into Kirlian photography in the United States. In the Kirlian process, developed in the Soviet Union, images are produced by electricity, rather than by light. Pictures are usually made while a subject rests his or her fingertips on the photographic plate, and some researchers believe the resulting picture reveals energy emanating from the person's hand.

Dr. Tiller was medium-built, in his early forties, and friendly. He took us to the off-campus home of a friend, where I was to work informally on a few people while hooked up to Kirlian equipment. The treatments went well, but the equipment, although among the finest available, malfunctioned, and Dr. Tiller was unable to obtain a useful, clear photograph. This didn't bother me, as there are many artifacts, such as dirt on your hands or fingers, the pressure applied by the hands onto the film, and static electricity, that often create false energy flairs. Also this equipment which supposedly measured energy was still in its developmental stage regarding its accuracy and reliability. Even then I realized that much more research will be needed to determine if Kirlian photography is an accurate method of measuring energy.

When we returned to the Stanford campus to drop off Dr. Tiller, we unexpectedly encountered Ted Bastin, who had devastating news. He had been discussing the results of the pendulum experiments with Hal Puthoff and Russell Targ, and the physicists had concluded that their controls for the tests had been inadequate. After I'd left, they had managed to stimulate a very slight signal, or spike, on the chart recorder by both of them jumping up and down right next to the bell jar and blowing hard on the pendulum case. As little as I knew about the scientific method, I knew controls were supposed to be checked *before* the trials.

This all sounded very peculiar and extremely unscientific to me, and when I talked later with Hal, he admitted that the signals produced by jumping and blowing were by no means as intense as the signals I had produced. He was well aware that I had been standing quietly eight or more feet from the pendulum. But, Hal said, if *any* signal, however small, could be produced artificially, SRI could not support the test results publicly, and no papers would be published on the experiment.

I was numb with anguish as Hal's words began to sink in. Publishing the results of experiments in respected journals is of the utmost importance in order to show the positive benefits of psychic testing.

At Judy's suggestion, we went to Noetic Sciences to see Brendan O'Regan, who would probably have more specific information and insight. One of Brendan's jobs at Noetics was to study experiments in parapsychology and evaluate their feasibility and possible ramifications.

I was nearly frantic as I told Brendan what had happened and that I wanted to replicate the pendulum experiment immediately, but this time under better controls. Brendan was sympathetic and tried to calm me, but I insisted that he contact Hal and Russell right away. I had to prove that I could affect their equipment under *any* controls they could devise. And it had to be tonight, for Rochelle and I were flying home to New York the next morning.

Brendan finally reached Russell, who said it would be impossible to return to the lab that night. Promptly, I offered to extend my stay and return to SRI on Thursday and Friday. But Puthoff's and Targ's schedules were already full for the next few weeks with a study of remote viewing, the ability to perceive distant places and objects psychically.

SRI, it seemed, at least on this occasion, was not really prepared to test and measure healing energy or even psychokinesis. In the next few hours I learned from Brendan that the pendulum experiment was actually part of Targ and Puthoff's remote viewing experiment—it had nothing at all to do with healing or PK research. Now everything finally made sense: This was just a haphazard attempt at a "look-see" of my skills. I wish I had been told this from the start, for I might not have felt so pressured.

I had come to California looking for corroboration of my abilities, expecting that science would provide answers to the questions I had about my gifts and this energy. I kept clinging to a sort of blind faith in the power of science, not realizing then that parapsychology research was still in its infancy. It occurred to me that perhaps I had expected too much from these experiments.

Before Rochelle and I left for New York, Judy invited several scientists who were receptive to working with me in the future to come to my hotel to get acquainted. First I met Henry Dakin, a plain, studious-looking man who was rather quiet and subdued, and young Jim Hickman, his tow-headed eager assistant, from the Dakin Labs in San Francisco. Impressed by what they had heard about me, they were interested in setting up a large-scale research schedule for me in April, five months away.

I told them about my first foray into the scientific method, but they seemed genuinely delighted with the results of my trip. This discussion with them made me feel less frustrated. Perhaps I had to be more patient, not one of my strong points.

When I met a physicist from Lawrence Livermore Laboratory, I was even more heartened. He wanted to arrange an April visit to a government-affiliated lab where I could participate in experiments to see whether I would be able to affect human cancer cells in test tubes. Now, this was what I wanted to do most of all—cancer research. After working with so many people who had the big C—and many of them successfully—I realized how important it would be to do this research. I truly believed that I could be instrumental in helping find a cure.

Knowing that I'd be returning to California for another chance to prove myself in more tightly regulated and controlled conditions placated my disappointment and gave me some reassurance. Maybe it was still possible for me to verify my healing ability and get significant test results published and accepted by the scientific community.

I was learning also that most scientists were suspicious of psychic phenomena, studies were atypical, and the results hard to duplicate. At that time, most researchers thought psychic research was an irritating subject, not worthy of serious attention, scrutiny, or funds. I might have shared such an attitude at one time, but now I was eager, almost desperate, to have my abilities gauged under their strict criteria.

All in all, though, my trip had been successful. I had met some good people in the field, and Rochelle and I had found time to reflect on our future and plan our lives together. We were appreciative for the trip and hoped only that the subsequent round would be even more fruitful. The next time I submitted myself to tests, I would be much better prepared, mentally and emotionally.

I could hardly wait.

8

In the Public Eye

One evening, Judy called to ask me if I would like to be on Barbara Walters's show *Not for Women Only.* She said the producer wanted me to participate in a panel discussion with some well-known people in the healing field. I quickly accepted. I was intrigued by some of the people who were to be on this panel—Dolores Krieger, a registered nurse who had started to teach other nurses "therapeutic touch" at New York University Hospital; and two well-known old-time faith/spiritual healers, Olga Worral and Ethel DeLoach.

When I arrived at the studio, I was introduced to Barbara Walters, and then, to my dismay, I saw Larry LeShan, my old nemesis. He was the psychologist-turned-psychic-healer who had discouraged me from trying to help people. We stopped short as we saw each other. He turned red as a beet, and I watched with concern as he walked angrily over to the show's producer. The subject of their discussion must have been me, for the next thing I knew, I was approached by the embarrassed producer. She said I could not be on the show, for it seemed LeShan had received a written invitation first. He was to be *the* psychic healer on the panel.

Of course I was offended and should have left the studio immediately. However, my adrenaline was high and I was curious as to the outcome of the show, so I sat in the audience and watched the program as a spectator. I was holding the lid down on my boiling irritation. The only one on the show whom I had any respect for was Ms. Krieger, and even she upset me because her opinion was that therapeutic touch, a form of the laying on of hands, was effective with only minor problems. She didn't believe this form of treatment could help serious conditions. And LeShan came off as defensive and pessimistic. It sounded like he didn't even believe in healing, yet he referred to himself as a "psychic healer" and even taught the subject.

Then, on December 23, 1974, the first major article about me was published in the *Village Voice,* a famous New York weekly. The front page of the paper carried a picture of me demonstrating my healing technique on Rochelle. A banner headline read, "The Brooklyn Healer," and in smaller letters were the words "Why the Psychics Are Betting on This Man," along with a separate editor's note on the cover, giving the paper's support of the authenticity of my abilities.

This article was an awakening, for, with my permission, the investigative reporter randomly chose one hundred case histories from my growing files. All the clients willingly spoke with the reporter, and I discovered that many had benefited from our work together, though they had never told me! When I expressed my surprise to them, they explained that when they saw their regular doctors and were helped, they never called to tell the doctors either. So I had a higher rate of success—85 percent, according to the reporter's calculations—than even I had imagined.

Coming as it did on the heels of my first research trip to California in my serious search for acceptance, the appearance of the article marked a victorious moment. Rochelle and I read the lengthy piece together, pleased to see how carefully written and accurate it was. The journalist, who had heard of me through Judy Skutch, surprised us with the thoroughness of his portrayal, which reported the events of my life up to that time and stressed the importance of my ability to demonstrate my powers in the laboratory.

Included in the article were interviews with many of my clients who had gone on the record about my work with them. Yoko Ono told how she had seen me perform PK in her apartment; a New York family-court judge confirmed that after my treatments he had experienced no more arthritis pain; and Buddy, Sam, and others told at length about the strange happenings that had taken place in Buddy's car.

That same week, the article John Peterson had written about my treatment of his back, which was better, and his knee tumor, which was now already smaller, appeared in the *National Observer.* That story, very conservative and low-key, was titled, "I'm Not Always Successful," a quote from me, and was a fine account of our session together.

I was delighted with the *Voice* and *Observer* articles, which I believed would lend credence to me personally, as well as to parapsychology. I did not anticipate that they would set off a virtual avalanche of secondary publicity. *Cosmopolitan* soon reprinted the *Voice* article, and suddenly newspapers and radio and television shows were fascinated—an ordinary guy who happily placed himself into the hands of scientific experts in order to validate his practicing the laying on of hands without religion, long robes, or mumbo jumbo.

In 1975 I had accepted my second invitation to appear on the *Pat Collins Show* on CBS, with Judy Skutch, spiritual healer Ethel DeLoach, and writer/physician William Nolen. Dr. Nolen had recently published a book: *Healing: In Search of a Miracle,* which was an account of his search for a case of true healing by such faith healers as the late Kathryn Kuhlman and Norbu Chen. His conclusion was that there was no evidence of people being cured by healers.

As I listened to Dr. Nolen I realized that he had investigated only healers who had never sought scientific and medical validations of their work. In fact, he wasn't aware that any healers had. So I brazenly asked if he would consider investigating me, a healer who subjected himself to the rigors of medical and scientific testing. He declined, thus confronted, but he did say that he thought healing powers do exist, though he had not yet run into any proven cases.

This incident with Nolen was disappointing and only confirmed the necessity of my appearing on respectable television and radio programs and giving select print interviews. More than ever the public needed to be fully and fairly informed about the validity of psychic healing.

I had no idea what was in store for me when author Dan Greenberg (*How to Be a Jewish Mother*) invited me to be on the Bill Boggs talk show in New York. I had already done Bill's show a while back, but Dan wanted me to go on with him this time because he was promoting his book on the paranormal. Unfortunately for Dan, he met me just days after his book had been published, witnessed my moving his ballpoint pen six feet across his parquet floor without ever touching it, and then was dismayed that he had just encountered the most amazing paranormal event in his entire life and it was not in his book. I felt bad—I liked Dan. So when he asked me to accompany him on some media events to tell the story of his PK experience with me, I agreed.

After my segment with Dan, I was flattered when Bill Boggs asked me to stay on for the rest of the show. But to my horror, out came an array of crystal-ball gazers, tarot-card readers wearing pointed hats, and witches and warlocks in full-costumed regalia.

I found myself trapped in the middle of a bizarre occult circus in front of millions of people! It was disconcerting to me that my scientifically oriented work was confused with that of these people. These were the types of people Dan had written about, but I didn't know this, for I hadn't yet read his book. If I had known I was going to be put into this mix, I never would have accepted. I was mortified and kept looking for ways to sneak off the stage. I found none but stayed far in the back, trying to disappear.

That show taught me a big lesson: Always find out who else is scheduled to be on a program, and never do anything like this again. I was angry at myself. How would I ever gain credibility for the laying on of hands if I was this naïve about media?

From now on I would not participate in every show or give interviews for all the articles that came my way. I would make media appearances only if I discerned them respectful of or educational about the subject of alternate healing. I insisted on taking the field of energy healing out of the occult basket.

On the other hand, all the media attention I received did have a positive effect. Already, countless people had had their minds opened, and many of the patients I have been able to help over the years might never have come to me were it not for the extensive coverage I received.

9

Battling Cancer

As I continued to practice healing, I began to appreciate the importance of understanding my patients' emotional states as well as their physical symptoms. I found that to most efficiently affect a disease, I had to work on more than the site of a problem, or the disease might emerge elsewhere in the body. If a section of your garden's soil is infected with insects or a fungus, you need to focus on not only that, but all the soil, lest it spread to other areas.

To root out an ailment, I found I had to work with a patient on mental, physical, and emotional levels. In order to do that I had to get to know and better understand each person and his or her environment. This treatment of the person as a whole is called "holistic healing."

I began to spend more time with my patients, getting more detailed pictures of their situations, as well as giving longer healing sessions—between fifteen and twenty minutes. I discovered that frequently, the more serious the ailment, the more treatments necessary to help heal it.

Now I had to protect myself even more, for I learned that serious illnesses were more draining than simple backaches or arthritis. I found that I needed to maintain a certain psychic distance from the people I worked with. Even as I opened my heart lovingly to my patients, I didn't want to open myself to disease on any level.

By far the more touching and distressing cases I take on are people with cancer. I always get caught on the roller coaster when I treat someone stricken with this world's-most-feared diagnosis. It is very difficult to get close to someone and have to watch him or her suffer through the ordeal and the underlying stigma of cancer. Your awareness of your own mortality is enormously heightened.

And should the cancer not respond to my efforts and get worse, I am a firsthand witness to the emotional and physical drain on the person and the family. We seem to forget that many chemotherapy treatments are still, even after thirty years, considered experimental. The doctors then knew even less than they do today about how to treat the plethora of cancers that have invaded our world.

Working with cancer is like waging a full-scale war. One day I win a battle, and the next I lose two—I feel like I'm battling doom. One factor that helped stoke my war on cancer was publicity. Along with word of mouth, it was through the mass media that more people and doctors started to learn of my newfound healing abilities.

I was fascinated when I learned from the writer of the *Village Voice* article that in the mid-1970s, New York City alone had more than one thousand laying-on-of-hands healers working quietly in fourth-floor walk-ups and out of view of the general public. But these other healers in New York and elsewhere did not subject themselves to the intensive scrutiny of medical and scientific investigation the way I did. Most worked with those suffering with lesser ailments, such as headaches. Few, if any, were keeping records and documenting their case histories—it was all done very informally, without consultations with the patients' doctors or written follow-ups.

Honestly, I found this hard to believe. How did these healers ever expect to raise the credibility and acceptance of alternative therapies in the

minds not only of the masses, but of the doctors and scientists, if they didn't keep details inscribed for posterity or do controlled experiments to discover the clinical effects their work had on these people? Weren't they even curious? Perhaps they were not concerned with these issues—I was consumed with them. Rarely did I have respect for and look upon another healer as a peer.

The torrent of publicity that poured down on me attracted many people seeking help with terminal cancer. I was deluged with rare and different forms of cancers I never before knew existed. My medical books quickly became dog-eared as I continually researched the manifestations and medical treatments of these different forms of cancer.

One particular cancer patient to whom I grew very close was Dan, a successful thirty-year-old graphic artist from New England. He seemed to have an enviable life—a beautiful wife, three healthy children, property, a good income—but his world had been shattered when his doctors told him he had a malignant brain tumor. The egg-sized growth was in the dominant hemisphere of his brain, and thus inoperable. Periodic X rays showed that the tumor was growing, creating increasing intracranial pressure and therefore precipitating grand mal seizures practically every day. Doctors had pronounced his death sentence—about three months to live.

When I first met Dan, I was pleased at how healthy he looked. Then he self-consciously removed his ski cap and wig for treatment, revealing that radiation therapy, administered in an attempt to shrink the tumor, had left him completely bald. But this was by far the least of his problems. Dan was also in deep emotional pain and very frightened.

"I know I have only three months left," he told me sadly that first day, "but I'm just not ready to leave my wife and kids!"

I felt helpless and uneasy, for I could not think of anything to say.

Dan's anger and frustration were surfacing.

"Damn it!" he cried. "I'm too young to die!" And I agreed.

He confessed that he'd lost faith in God, and I was pained when he told me how lonely he felt—the loneliness of being "different." Unable

to face their own fears of death, Dan's friends had virtually abandoned him and his family. My heart went out to him.

His desperation was palpable, and, wanting to be of help, I began the treatment. Concentrating on Dan's brain condition, I focused on a clear, sharp image, as if I had suddenly switched on a television set. I "saw" a two-inch oval tumor in what looked like a spongy substance. Then I visualized my energy, like shimmering heat flickering from a burning candle, radiating into the spongy surrounding area and into the tumor itself. Then I imagined the tumor shriveling and becoming smaller. I strongly believed that the growth would waste away as I exerted my own willpower to try to help him. My tenacious confidence spurred me on.

When I was finished, Dan told me he had felt as if some unusual activity were taking place in his head, specifically the area where the tumor was, though of course, he was quick to stipulate he couldn't be sure. I too felt certain that I had made contact, but the results of Dan's next X rays would be the proof of the pudding. A patient's subjective reports are always important, but more important are the impartial results of medical tests.

I worked intensively with Dan a couple of times a week for the next three weeks, and then he was X-rayed. His brain tumor had decreased to half its original size—the inside of it looked as if it had disintegrated, like it had been burned away. The doctors could not explain the unforeseen change, nor could they explain the corresponding disappearance of Dan's daily seizures or his renewed sense of hope.

As I continued to work with Dan, we became friends. For my birthday he gave me a double-volume set of *Harrison's Principles of Internal Medicine.* He was a strikingly intelligent young man, very scientifically oriented, and I learned a lot from him during our time together.

After six months, Dan's cancerous tumor shrank to a pinhead of scar tissue and Dan was finally able to return to work. But there was a flip side—he stopped seeing Rochelle and me on the friendly, social basis we had established during the time I had worked with him. Regretably, I

took his withdrawal very personally, for I thought perhaps it was because we came from different social backgrounds—Dan was a member of a very wealthy and distinguished family—and he no longer needed me.

After a few months of silence I received a long letter. In it Dan explained that he still cared strongly for Rochelle and me, but that seeing me reminded him of the black days when he was planning his funeral and updating his will. I came to understand his need to leave behind the painful memories that had become indistinguishably linked with me.

It was becoming evident to Rochelle and me that making and keeping friends would be difficult undertakings. What most people take for granted was a rarity in our already unique lives. People were either too intimidated to see beyond "the healer" or too envious of my abilities. If only they could see through my eyes . . .

Peter Gimbel, the producer of the extraordinarily successful documentary *Blue Water, White Death,* whom Dan recommended me to, came to see me about a small circular growth over his left eyebrow. His doctor had diagnosed the six-month growth as a basal cell carcinoma, a skin cancer, and a biopsy was scheduled.

Though such growths generally can be treated quite successfully by doctors, Peter was terribly alarmed by the doctor's diagnosis. My first impulse was to try to calm him. Then I worked locally on his forehead. About three days later, Peter called with astonishing news—the small cancerous growth had simply fallen off! It had virtually popped out of his skin. His doctors were stunned—this just did not happen—but examination showed the skin over Peter's brow to be normal.

Even with my expanding workload, I still made housecalls. It was a bright, sunny day when Rochelle and I walked into a ritzy apartment building in New York's swank Upper East Side. We were there to see the famous singer Ethel Merman at the behest of her son. It was not publicly known then, but Ethel had brain cancer and was quickly losing her fight. The doctors had been able to remove only a small piece of the tumor, and declared it was not enough for a cure. Her prognosis was terminal. She too was completely bald from her chemical therapy, but this no longer impressed me. Sadly, I was becoming used to seeing this common ill effect of chemotherapy and radiation treatments.

After introductions, I began to work on this vulnerable woman whom I'd seen on television countless times. What I remember most about our visits was that Ethel would hum and swing her arms while I treated her, conducting to the sounds and rhythms of my energy she alone heard clearly.

I worked with her weekly for a number of weeks, and her next X ray showed that her brain tumor had shrunk in size by more than 50 percent! I was delighted with this improvement. But my enthusiasm was short-lived—I learned from her son that a family doctor/friend suggested she undergo the first rounds of a brand-new experimental chemotherapy treatment. She was to be the first human recipient—the decision had been made.

I was very confused by this decision, since my work seemed to be having a beneficial effect. But I realized I could not help her while she was having this new chemotherapy treatment and resigned reluctantly from the case.

It was a month later when I received a letter from the son telling me his mom had died. He wrote that the only time she'd received any positive benefit was when she was working with me. A 50-percent reduction of an unremovable tumor incredibly was created solely by my ministrations.

I wished this made me feel better, but it didn't—cancer can create terrible confusion—especially when one has to make decisions for someone else.

Ethel Merman's situation was not really unusual. Perhaps I would have done exactly the same as her son had, but I believe each case is individual and no one can pass judgment on a family for doing what they sincerely believe to be the best for their loved one.

When young Helen Moreno came to see me, she had cancer of the cervix, revealed by a cone biopsy, and a fibroid tumor. Her doctors had told Helen, a public school teacher in her late forties, to prepare herself for a complete hysterectomy. Even though she had no intentions of having another child, she was terrorized by the thought. When she and I discussed her illness, it emerged that Helen had consulted with only one physician. I wanted her to get a second opinion. So before I even began working with her, I referred her to a gynecologist with whom I had worked previously. His diagnosis, however, was the same as that of the first doctor—a complete hysterectomy would give Helen the best chance of recovery.

With Helen I worked above the area of her pelvis where the tumor was located, and visualized its demise. About a month later, she returned to her first doctor at Flower Fifth Avenue Hospital in Manhattan. To the doctor's astonishment, the fibroid tumor was gone and Helen's Pap smear was normal—there was no longer any need for a hysterectomy. The second doctor ran the same tests and arrived at the same conclusion—she had been healed. I believe that second and even third opinions are absolutely essential and often life-saving steps to ascertain that the correct diagnosis has been given.

Another lady that stands out in my mind is Adela Carney, whose mother and stepfather were prominent social figures in San Antonio, Texas. They had heard about my work from one of the private funders of Stanford Research Institute's parapsychology research. A petite girl in her early twenties, Adela looked like a skeleton when she was helped into my office by her mother and her aunt, who supported her on either side. Her clothes were hanging loosely off her, and she was so pale that she was almost ghostly.

When Adela was four months pregnant with her second child, a cyst on her right ovary was diagnosed, and during surgery, cancer was discovered. Both ovaries and tubes were removed, but Adela refused to let her growing fetus be removed and even turned down chemotherapy and radiation treatments until after the child's birth. The doctors expected the baby to spontaneously abort but it did not.

Twenty-four hours after her baby boy was born, an exploratory operation was performed and, unfortunately, the cancer had spread to the kidneys, liver and stomach. The surgeons removed what they could, closed her up, and dispensed radiation and chemo, but the prognosis was dire—the doctors did not give her much time.

This is when her mother demanded Adela see me. By the time she came to see me she could hardly walk. She vomited blood nearly every day and could not hold down food. Her doctors had given up—they said Adela had at most three weeks to live—so Adela and her family had traveled to my office in Brooklyn. When I looked at this ashen, bony woman, I believed her doctors might be right.

I carefully explained to the three women that I had worked with cancer before, sometimes with good results, but that I could not promise or guarantee any improvement of any kind. I assured them, however, that I would do the very best in my power to try to help her.

Adela lay on the recliner, and I sat behind her, closed my eyes, and blanked out everything around me—the whir of the air conditioner, the soft buzz of voices from the crowded waiting room, the almost palpable anxiety of the two older women.

As I lowered my left hand to her mid-back and placed my right hand on her forehead, she shuddered. When I moved my right hand two inches above the top of her head, I realized her skin was clammy, and her breathing was shallow. She also had an odor similar to that of other dying people I had worked with.

Not allowing myself to be emotionally affected, I tried to stimulate her "lifeline," willing my thoughts toward hope and encouragement, not death. I wanted Adela to respond, to improve! And she would need to do so quickly, for I could almost *feel* this ravaging disease eating her up inside. I could actually sense a resistant force very similar to that between magnetic polar opposites.

I was becoming very drained, as though her cancer were trying to squeeze the life out of me. After about twenty minutes, I lifted my hands and pushed the recliner forward. Adela had a relaxed and contented smile on her face and, to everyone's shock, she briskly got up from the recliner and prepared to leave without assistance from her mom and aunt.

Adela and her family came to the office every day for the rest of the week, and Adela looked better each time. Her yellowed complexion, jaundiced as a result of her liver's involvement in her cancer, was turning a rosier color, and there was a sparkle in her eyes when she told me of the improvements she'd experienced. Her appetite had returned—after our first session she could hardly wait to get to a restaurant, where she greedily consumed a cheeseburger, french fries, and a chocolate milk shake. This had impressed Adela's mother most of all, because until then she'd practically had to force-feed her.

On the last day of her treatment, Adela, looking wonderful, almost bounced into the office. As I lightly touched her shoulders, I felt her energy level had begun to normalize, and she was no longer vacuuming the energy from me. The thought that she was definitely improving flashed through my mind.

Before seeing me, Adela had complete blood tests done and when she returned home six days later, the tests were repeated. The doctors could not believe the difference in her white blood count—they were amazed. The following week she went camping in Tennessee with her two boys and husband, something her doctors kept saying was out of the question, that she would never live through it. And I received a postcard two weeks later from Tennessee. "Thank you," it read. "Having a wonderful time."

Over the next year I conducted several series of treatments on Adela, sometimes in San Antonio, sometimes in New York. I always looked forward to seeing the weight she'd gained, the fullness of her once-gaunt face, and the restored luster of her pale blond hair.

Then, unexpectedly, two years after our first sessions together, Adela's mother called me from a hospital in San Antonio and told me that Adela had undergone exploratory surgery. I became very distraught, but Adela's mother quickly explained that Adela had demanded the surgery—she so strongly believed that the cancer was completely gone from her body that she wanted confirmation from her surgeon. Adela's doctor had advised against the operation, and for good reasons—he feared that if there were cancer cells anywhere around the incision, the surgery itself might stimulate their growth and cause them to spread. But Adela had insisted—she was a tough cookie. She was out of surgery, and within hours the doctors had found no trace of the cancer. It was a drastic action, but I had to admit that the results were miraculous, both for her sake and as a confirmation of her healing.

As Adela's mother spoke, I joyfully envisioned Adela fully restored to health and surrounded by her two beautiful sons.

Around that same time, I began work with Sharon Dwyer on a malignant lesion in her eye. Soon after, the lesion had disappeared. I encouraged her to continue what I call "maintenance" treatment—when someone gets well, I like to taper off their sessions and eventually see the person only for infrequent follow-ups to help keep their body strong. However, she led a full and busy life and found it difficult to get to New York on any sort of schedule.

Unfortunately, a couple years later, I was called to Lenox Hill Hospital in Manhattan to try once again to help this thirty-eight-year-old woman who had a sudden reoccurrence of cancer. This situation was even more unusual for me—Sharon was in a coma. Her surgeon believed she might die within hours. Her cancer, which had first developed in her breasts, had metastasized further, spreading throughout her body and into her spine and brain. Before she'd drifted into the little-known, eerie world of coma, increased brain pressure had brought on seizures. Her husband, Steven, remembered how effective I had been originally with Sharon, and called me in a final grasp at a miracle.

I worked fervently with Sharon in the hospital for two days, trying to waken her sleeping consciousness but without getting through. We saw no encouraging changes. Her surgeon and all the nurses knew who I was, and at her husband's and my request, my treatments were noted on Sharon's chart, along with medication, temperature, blood pressure, and brain-wave information.

When Sharon's condition continued to decline, her doctor told her husband to send for the family so they could say good-bye. Steven called me again, although by now all he really hoped for was that I would be able to energize Sharon enough so that she would come out of the coma long enough to see her children a final time. But I wanted so much more for her.

At the hospital, as I approached Sharon's room, I saw the chief surgeon emerging from his office. He had been introduced to me previously by Sharon's family, and had accepted my participation in her case graciously and openly. Now he carefully explained her condition to me.

"Look," he concluded, "the fact is that if she can even come out of her coma now, it would be a miracle. So go see what you can do." And he turned and walked down the quiet hall with tears in his eyes, for he had been Sharon's doctor and friend for many years.

Sharon's husband and teenaged daughter were waiting to see her. I asked them to give me about twenty minutes. As I sat in Sharon's room beside the bed, facing this frail, once very attractive woman, I took her limp hand in mine. And I was driven to attempt something I never had before—to go deep into the recesses of her mind and into the coma state with her. I realized it seemed a bit radical, and didn't even know if it could be done, but I desperately wanted to help her. Understanding that many coma patients are still somewhat conscious but cannot communicate, I decided to try to speak with her telepathically, silently, mind-to-mind.

This was unexplored territory, but somehow I felt guided, though still fearful of this strange undertaking. Automatically I began my long, slow breaths to calm myself. Then I spoke in my mind directly to Sharon: "Sharon, it's Dean. Remember me? Sure you do. If you can hear me, squeeze my hand." After several minutes I realized there was no response—her hand lay quietly in mine.

Again I took a few more deep breaths, closed my eyes, and allowed my hands to move, one on her forehead and one just below her neck. I began trying to "pump" her up, like doing CPR with energy—to connect with her essential life force, her spirit, her soul, anything.

I do not do it very often, but sometimes when I'm involved in a particularly difficult cancer case, I ask for help, and I did so that day. I looked into myself, reaching up into that inner Source that connects us all with the universe, and I said a prayer of my own: "Please, help me. Please, help this young woman live!"

Immediately after saying those words to myself, I felt something very strange happen. I saw, as if from a distance, an amazing aura of lights, a visible vibrating energy around my body. And with that, a sudden rush of wind seemed to fill my ears. I felt myself propelled through an astounding tube of swirling patterns of bright lights that rushed past me, pulled into some type of wind tunnel, a dimension where there was no physical body, only a "floating mind." The whirlwind was hauling my mind through the brightness toward a quieter, darker, eerie depth of moving stars and space, a nebula of a cyclone of clouds, light, and matter. I seemed to have entered an expanding vortex. Darkness lay ahead, and I knew intuitively that I had to stay within the brightness. I don't know how I knew this, but I did.

I had a brief moment of trepidation. I hesitated, and then a blast of wind plunged me into this twister, this sideways tornado. Then suddenly I saw a figure of blue lights that I felt was Sharon's energy body. I pursued her pale lightbody in this awesome whirling mass. In spite of my determination to catch up to her, it was slow going, uphill against a raging wind, and I was petrified. Where the hell was I? Had I actually joined Sharon in her comatose state?

Telepathically I called out to Sharon, "Wait for me, I am coming to get you." I was rushing down this bright tunnel toward her faint blue translucent lightform that seemed a far distance ahead. And beyond Sharon's energy form, it looked like the amazing lights were widening at the mouth of this unusual vortex and metamorphosing into the endless expanse of blackness and stars. I had to prevent Sharon from going into the darkness.

In my mind, I yelled to her, "Come back. . . . Sharon . . . don't go. . . . Come back toward the light." An echoey tone that sounded like her voice filled my mind: "Where am I? . . ." Was she actually communicating with me through thought-transference? I could only hope so.

"Sharon, try to move toward me. . . . I can't seem to catch up to you. . . . You must try to come to me. . . . Will yourself . . ." my mind now whispered.

Her flickering lightbody seemed to hover, undecided, then continued drifting closer to what seemed to be the border of an abyss.

"I feel like I'm being pulled . . ." I thought I heard Sharon say.

I could not believe what was happening to me, and though I had no idea of what to do next, I decided to reach out and grab her from where she seemed perilously close to that edge, the irislike entrance to the dark tunnel, the separator of life and death. In a flash, my own energy body enveloped hers and pulled her away.

"Come with me, Sharon. You are safe with me. . . ." I thought.

"Where to? . . ." was the faint response.

"Back to the bright white light behind us . . . Back to your family . . ." I answered in my mind.

The vivid lights grew more brilliant as together we struggled through an even heavier turbulence that threatened to tear us apart. I felt like a lifeguard trying to tow an unconscious swimmer through a raging sea. Abruptly we were back in the hospital room, and I was collapsed in my chair, my head pounding ferociously, just like when I did PK.

Suddenly it was as if Sharon had been touched by an electric probe. Her body jerked, and her eyes opened. I absorbed this movement through a cloudy haze and slowly made my own return to the reality of the intensive care unit. It had been extraordinary! Sharon looked at me with a smile, and her eyes twinkled with tears and understanding. We both knew what we had been through, and there was no need for words.

Within minutes, Steven and Sharon's daughter entered the room. They almost passed out when they saw her struggling to sit up in her bed, and hurried forward to assist her. I didn't want her to lose the strength she had so suddenly gained. So, though still groggy, I slowly stood up, placed one hand on the back of Sharon's neck, and concentrated on pummeling loving energy into her body, while she and her family huddled together, weeping. I was overwhelmed and had to stay a while longer in order to recuperate and regain my composure.

The following morning, the chief surgeon, who had left the hospital before I'd finished treating Sharon, went into her room, expecting the worst. I was told he was flabbergasted when Sharon got out of bed and walked across the room to him, unsteadily but with astounding determination.

"What's up, Doc?" she said, her sense of humor obviously having returned along with her sudden readmission to the real world. I was told the doctor almost fainted.

The day before, X rays made of Sharon's brain tumor had revealed large cancerous lesions. The day after she came out of the coma, new X rays showed that the cancer was gone. Gone! I was accustomed to cancer cases where a tumor grew progressively smaller over a period of time, but this was a real bull's-eye!

Two weeks later, Sharon left the hospital, and per the family's request, Rochelle and I traveled to their ranch in Pennsylvania, where we stayed about a week so I could continue working with Sharon. On that Easter Sunday, she got up, said hello to her family, and walked slowly to the stable to see her other loves, her horses.

When I finally allowed myself the space to think about that incredible and shocking coma expedition, I still found it hard to fully comprehend. I knew that what I had been through was not a dream. It was all too real—the telepathy, the flash of racing lights, the powerful surging of wind rushing through me, and Sharon's comeback. Then the realization hit me: This disquieting sojourn had unknowingly taken me to the vortex between life and death. I felt like a reluctant astronaut exploring new worlds of inner space.

I began to realize how crucial timing is in healing and that numerous variables—my energy level and mental state, the patient's energy and mental condition, the position of the moon and sun, the electromagnetic and gravitational forces around the earth, and more—all contribute to the healing. These factors have to line up, like multiple sights on a gun. When they are in a perfect row, that's when I believe "real" magic can happen—the instant miracle!

This time I had been successful. What would happen if I didn't succeed next time? Could I get stuck on the other side of this vortex, never to return? Maybe die?

When I first met Carl Woolf, I knew I had encountered a unique situation. Carl had been fighting multiple myeloma, a cancer of the bone marrow, for an unbelievable twelve years, and he was now experiencing the roughest period since his illness struck. His long struggle proved that the body can fight cancer, but now, except for an occasional excursion in a wheelchair, he was confined to a hospital bed. His immunological system was at a very low point, and he was quite weak, but his doctors had decided to allow him to go home. There was nothing left for them to try, and they felt he should die in the comfort of familiar surroundings, with his family nearby.

Multiple myeloma can create multiple fractures and intense pain. There were times when Carl would make a simple ordinary movement and a bone would break. It was rapidly becoming almost impossible for him to move at all. Even his attempts to smile were full of agony, because he was depressed by the unrelenting pain, nausea, and the appetite and weight loss that accompanied his disease. He earnestly told me that he no longer cared about living, and wanted to die. There was more readiness than fear on his part.

Before coming to me, Carl had tried virtually every available therapy, conventional and alternative. He had been referred by a medical doctor who had practiced acupuncture, and had explored other alternate healing methods. Traditional medicine, acupuncture, hypnosis, psychiatry, homeopathy, and chiropractology had not helped Carl.

I focused every bit of energy I could on destroying the cancer cells in Carl's bones, and after several treatments within two weeks, he felt so unusually well that he invited his old card-playing gang to his house, where he sat for many hours engrossed in playing poker. Carl's attitude changed, and now he would plead with me to try to save him—he no longer wanted to die.

During the next few sessions, I kept my attention on killing the cancer, and also visualized less pain and a stronger lifeline. I continued to see healing energy waves entering his bones, enriching the blood, and destroying the cancer.

Within days, Carl was able to leave the prison of his bed. At times, to our shock and elation, he was able to walk about on his own, without the dreaded wheelchair. His skeletal pain diminished, the nausea subsided, and his appetite improved. After six months of daily consumption, he was able to stop taking addictive narcotics. In the first month I treated him, he gained more than seven pounds, and we were very encouraged.

But suddenly, after nearly six months of such heartening progress, Carl began an alarming decline. Although I overextended myself and worked diligently with him almost every day, I felt him slipping back into the familiar fatigue. Gratefully there was one conspicuous difference—he had absolutely no pain whatsoever.

Carl reentered the hospital, and within forty-eight hours, he fell into a coma. I desperately tried to connect with the now elusive thread of his lifeline, that little "tingle" of energy I was able to sense that told me everything. But no matter how intense my concentration, no matter how much it mattered to me personally to save him, I believed his soul and vital life forces were already beginning to separate from the almost lifeless, diseased mass of brittle bone and thin flesh that was his body, and transcend.

Suddenly Carl's eyes popped open. He was wide awake, lucid, and his expression was filled with tranquillity. Abruptly stronger, he grabbed my hand, pulled me closer to him, and whispered, "God bless you for everything, Dean. It's a wonderful feeling to be ready."

Carl closed his eyes and gently returned to the coma, but now I couldn't stop myself—I had to try in spite of his words. With untapped determination, I closed my eyes, took a deep breath, and forced myself to enter that strange turbulent tunnel of lights and sounds, the maelstrom of the vortex.

And amazingly, I found I could will myself there! My experience was similar to the first time in which I had attempted to bring someone back from the precipice, but when I saw a glowing lightbody that had to be Carl floating far ahead of me, somehow I knew it was going to be different.

Growing fainter by the second, Carl's dim energy form was already beyond the iris that was opening and closing in the shadowed area beyond. His feeble lightform was already past the huge, swirling opening ahead, but I attempted to pursue him anyway. In my mind, I silently shouted, "Carl . . . can you hear me? . . ."

"Dean? . . . Where am I? . . ." I heard him question.

"Don't go any farther. . . . Wait for me, Carl. . . . I want to bring you back. . . ." I thought desperately.

"No . . . no need . . ." I heard faintly.

Then the deafening noise! I could barely hear myself think! The tremendous thundering like a speeding train coming toward me . . . The churning radiance of lights distracting me from my objective, flashing wildly and blinding me. Then a sudden silence, as if we were in the brief quiet of the eye of a hurricane.

"Dean . . . this is my time to go home . . . and I am ready. . . . You must go back. . . . Still so much you have to do . . ." The faint whispering of Carl's thoughts ravaged me as much as the roaring tunnel had a moment ago. I was consumed with Carl's thoughts. The last thing I heard was "Thank you, Dean. . . . Words cannot express my gratitude . . ." and then the pale form far ahead of me suddenly burst into a fireworks of beautiful magnificence. In an immediate rush, I felt myself tumbling and plummeting back through this extraordinary tunnel—alone.

Instantly, I found myself at Carl's bedside, laying across his now slack body, still holding his lifeless hand tightly within mine. Even though I knew he had transcended, the peace that totally encompassed my own being felt so pure and overpowering, I could not question the tranquillity he must have felt in his passage back "home." It felt right.

Regardless of my zeal, I realized that the decision between life and death was not mine to make, but I knew it was part of my mission to try to keep people alive to allow them the greatest opportunity to recover. I had been given a wonderful and precious gift, but it was not always in my control, not even when it mattered most to me.

When a soft-spoken voice teacher from upstate New York, Sarah Fisher, began seeing me for treatments, we established a special rapport because of our shared love for music. Sarah came to me when she was recuperating from a double radical mastectomy. Her surgery had been to no avail, for the doctors had discovered substantial lymph node involvement and the cancer was already spreading to Sarah's lungs and liver.

Sarah was very weak because of the radiation and chemotherapy administered to her. I was maintaining a hectic schedule, trying to help everyone that sought me out, and more frequently I was called out of town. When I had to leave patients like Sarah, even briefly, I felt terribly torn.

Sarah, who understood my torment, was always advising me to slow down: "Dean, you can't heal the whole world—you're only one person."

One day she brought me a card on which she'd meticulously printed a quote from the Talmud: "He who sustains one life is regarded as if he had created the world."

This excerpt helped me gain some perspective on the frantic life I was leading and made me consider the need to pace myself to avoid burnout.

During a year of treatments with me, Sarah responded dramatically well. Her pain lessened, and her breathing difficulties went away. But then she grew weak again, and the cancer began to overwhelm her body. I fought the dreaded disease with all my might and continued working with her in the hospital. But again, the miracle I wanted so desperately did not come.

I have come to realize that death is an ever-looming presence. It is a part of life. When a patient dies, I feel a personal loss, and the length of time during which I knew her or him made no difference. Even if I knew the person only a short while, my connection was strong and exclusive. Special.

But I've also come to realize that sometimes death *is* the healing, especially when the patient is suffering interminably and nothing traditional or holistic is helping.

The intensive work necessary with cancer patients helped give me an introduction to the role the mind can play in the development of disease. It alarmed me that a common thread ran through a number of the medically terminal cancer patients I saw. Besides the people genetically predisposed to disease, many had become ill within a short time after a major emotional upheaval, such as the loss of a loved one, the collapse of a career, the breakup of a marriage, or some other traumatic event. Somehow, mental and emotional stress had manifested itself into physical illness.

I strongly believed then, as I do now, that it is imperative that people worldwide be informed of this one single piece of potentially lifesaving information. This knowledge in itself can help people start to control their own lives and reduce the stress they are under, thus preventing the apparent chain reaction from automatically taking over.

Now new questions hounded me: If the human mind is strong enough to create disease, can the same mind help banish illness and produce good health? What kind of guidance and discipline would assist and enable people to achieve this? Especially people ridden with cancer—they need to focus every ounce of their energy in helping themselves.

These questions definitely stimulated me into trying an unusual experiment on myself. I'd had a medium-sized wart on my right middle finger for many years. I was a little self-conscious about it, and to my dismay, the wart suddenly began to grow larger. Some doctors say warts are the by-products of a systemic viral dysfunction, so I thought that if I could help stimulate someone else's immune system, then I should be able to activate my own healing mechanism and dissolve the growth.

My focus was to shrink the growth and raise the level of my immune system so the wart would not come back. I chose a quiet room where I would be undisturbed, lay down on a couch, and got myself comfortable. Then I closed my eyes, did a few body stretches, took several deep breaths, and tried to blank out all outside thoughts and stresses.

Suddenly, an image appeared in my mind. It was a white outline of my body. A four-inch-wide bluish-white band of light started to travel from the top of my head and down the left side of my body, encircling the perimeter of this image. It generated a warm feeling as it moved. It was interesting, for this bright light and warmth seemed to be related to and propelled by my breathing pattern. As I inhaled, the band of light moved slowly, and as I exhaled, it moved more quickly.

This illumination continued on its tour around my body's image—around my legs and the right side of my body, then back to the top of my head. Then it began another revolution.

After this band of healing light revolved around my body image several times, I then noticed that as it reached my right hand and middle finger, the light grew wider, almost twice the original width, and even more vibrant. My finger felt not only warmer but almost hot as the brilliant light passed over the area. While the light was on my hand and finger, I consciously visualized the wart getting smaller. Then the light decreased to its previous size as it made several more rotations in the same manner. Each time the light and soothing warmth passed over my right hand and finger, it expanded.

After about fifteen minutes I felt satisfied with my initial attempt to shrink this growth. Instinctively, as with my healing work, I felt that doing this only once would not be enough, so I repeated the same process daily over the next week. Soon, the wart that had been on my finger for years and had recently started growing was now much smaller. Each day it appeared to be dissolving. After another few days, to my delight, the growth was gone.

This experiment stimulated my curiosity and imagination about other possibilities, and I began to develop a combination of different imaging techniques—not only for self-healing but also that others could use. I tried them out on a number of people, including a few interested and innovative medical doctors and psychologists. I was very encouraged when one medical doctor, whose own physician had nothing to offer but pain medication, reported that he was finally able to alleviate his lower back pain, which had been bothering him for years.

There were a number of others in this first group who also were successful in relieving their own painful conditions, such as headaches, premenstrual syndrome, stomach cramps, leg cramps, and even adverse side effects of chemotherapy like nausea and fatigue. Some of them were helping themselves with more than one problem! After receiving this constructive feedback, I believed I had made a giant step into a relatively unknown area of teaching people how to help themselves.

It was 1975 when Rochelle and I organized and conducted my first public "Self-Help and Laying-on-of-Hands Seminar" in Brooklyn, New York. There were more than two hundred people in attendance at this large Knights of Columbus hall. We had a diversified group that included patients of mine, psychologists, medical doctors, lay people, scientists, and friends.

I started everybody off with a physical destressing technique, teaching them how to breath properly and to release the physical stress in their bodies. Then I followed with a mental destressing exercise, having them visualize a peaceful scene, like a lake setting, and blanking out all thoughts that came in as ripples on their clear, smooth body of water.

Next I guided them through my body-circulation technique, which I developed after visualizing the white band of light that shrunk my wart. I always let the people know that if they have health problems they should see that white light expand to double its width over and into the problem area. Then they should visualize a close-up of that problem and focus healing waves of energy flowing into the troublesome region.

Afterward I paired the group off and shared some of my laying-on-of-hands methods that they could try on their loved ones. The seminar was a great success, and in the months that followed, many of the participants gave me excellent feedback on how they helped themselves with certain health problems and how they were able to release their everyday stresses. A number of the medical doctors, psychologists, and laypeople told me stories of how they had helped others through my laying-on-of-hands techniques.

I followed up with other seminars across the United States and came to the obvious conclusion that, to a certain degree, we all can positively affect our own bodies, as well as others', by doing specific mental visualizations. These seminars activated me into further developing my own theories and methods especially tailored to my patients with cancer and other illnesses. These ailing people could not rely just on outside help—I believed they had to work on themselves and participate in their own healing.

I knew also that with the support and encouragement of medical doctors, people would start taking self-help and preventative measures more seriously and that, eventually, self-help techniques would be a regular supplement to other traditional and holistic approaches. A new focus and path was beginning to beckon me.

10

Scientific Testing:

A Successful Second Round

FINALLY IT WAS TUESDAY, APRIL 15, 1975, THE day after my twenty-fifth birthday. At five o'clock in the morning I was lying in a spacious bed at the Burlingame Hyatt House in San Francisco, looking on with envy as Rochelle slept. I couldn't sleep anymore—I couldn't stop thinking. The rising sun signaled that my second attempt at scientifically proving my healing abilities was about to begin. In a few hours I would start a ten-day battery of tests, which I hoped would result in more definitive information than the first tests I had undergone. I felt the pressure on me steadily increasing.

Submitting myself to the tests was not a completely selfless act for the benefit of science. *I* was the curious one. I still needed answers to the same old questions: Did I in fact produce energy that healed? What kind of energy was it? Where did it come from? Why me? I was sure that the better I understood the energy I channeled, the better I would be able to direct and focus it to help people with their illnesses. This was my crusade.

I also wanted to learn all I could about the equipment, procedures, and controls utilized in proper research into parapsychological phenomena. Since our first visit to California, Rochelle and I had begun to discuss establishing our own research foundation. I hoped that during this trip I would learn enough so that when the time came, I would be able to guide my own organization into better-controlled paranormal research.

The alarm clock shocked me out of my reverie.

Through Judy's intercession, this trip had been underwritten by Henry Dakin, a wealthy electrophysicist and inventor, who had paid Rochelle's and my airfare, a fee for my time, and fees to a variety of labs and academic institutions that would be participating in the study. Henry was one in a close-knit group of scientists I'd already met who worked with Judy and the Institute of Noetic Sciences in testing sensitive subjects. Several years before, he had converted his old brownstone house, situated in one of the lovely residential sections of San Francisco, into a highly sophisticated, multifloored laboratory for parapsychology research and for the development of his own inventions. Today was my orientation day at Dakin Laboratories—the tests would begin tomorrow.

Assistant researchers Jim Hickman and Roger Macdonald, both about thirty, gave Rochelle and me a tour of the lab. Then Henry Dakin, a gray-haired somber man in his late forties, greeted us. Henry was pleasant but somewhat distant, as though he were preoccupied with other business, and Jim didn't seem as open and eager as he had been when I met him during my first California trip. They both were polite but seemed to be holding me at arm's length. At first I thought it was their way of maintaining scientific objectivity, but later Judy told me that Dakin had been annoyed and upset about some recent articles published about me, particularly one in a sensational tabloid. Judy advised me to ignore Jim's and Henry's coolness, for she believed, as I did, that publicity was important in educating the public. I just hoped their attitudes wouldn't affect the publication of any test results.

As Jim, Roger, Rochelle, and I walked through the corridors of Dakin

Labs, Jim explained some of the experiments involved in our study. The project was called "Preliminary Physical Measurements of Psychophysical Effects Associated with Three Alleged Psychic Healers"—quite a mouthful. Also participating in the study were faith healers Olga Worrall and the Reverend John Scudder. Reverend Scudder had already completed his tests, and Mrs. Worrall would be tested after me. I found it interesting that even the scientists confused psychic, or energy, healers with faith healers—if they weren't clear on the difference, how could the public be? To me, faith meant religion—psychic meant energy healing, in which one need not believe in any religion to be helped.

In a number of the experiments we would attempt to replicate work done previously by notable parapsychology researchers. Some of these replications were to deal with electric and magnetic field variations, others with plant growth and brain-wave measurements.

As my first day at Dakin Labs drew to a close, Jim and Roger handed me the schedule for the next nine days. Some of my tests would be conducted elsewhere, at a number of government and university-affiliated research centers and institutes in the area. The next day would include brain-wave work at Stanford Research Institute, and an experiment on a hypertensive laboratory rat at a medical institute. The rest of the week I would be based at Dakin Labs. The following week would include an alluring experiment with HeLa cancer cells in test tubes at Lawrence Livermore Laboratory. It would be a heavy workload, but I felt eager and ready to begin.

Wednesday morning, Rochelle and I were driven to SRI. Though I would not be seeing Targ and Puthoff on this trip, I was going to work again with Dr. Erik Peper of the biomedical department. This time he was going to monitor my brain waves and those of a volunteer "patient" during a healing session. He hoped to establish a correlation between my healing-state brain-wave patterns and those of the recipient.

Dr. Peper explained that I would treat the volunteer in an electrically shielded room, which was separated from the room where the scientists monitored their machines, by what looked like a two-foot-thick refrigerator door. In the "treating room," both the volunteer and I would be wired to an EEG, she reclining in a lounge chair and I sitting in a club chair behind her. Jim Hickman would remain in the room as an observer. Rochelle and Roger Macdonald would be allowed to observe from the outer room.

Dr. Peper, Jim, and I talked while they started the tedious and messy procedure of attaching the EEG wires to different parts of my head with that awful sticky paste. Then Dr. Peper introduced the volunteer and attached wires to her head in the same way. We were given careful instructions. If, during the session, I felt I had reached a peak in my healing state, I was to press a button on the chair arm to indicate this to Peper. If the woman felt herself in a state of unusually deep relaxation, she was to press a similar button.

Dr. Peper showed us an intercom system that would enable us to communicate with him once he went into the next room. Then he, Rochelle, and Macdonald exited and closed the thick door, leaving Jim, the volunteer, and me in the treating room.

Over the intercom, Dr. Peper told us to continue talking casually—he wanted to record our normal, or baseline, brain waves. Then he told me to begin the actual healing. I automatically sank into a deep tranquil state and focused on a general relaxation treatment for the volunteer. Gradually I felt myself achieving a balance between my mind and my body—I felt blissful. Then I remembered the button. I removed one hand from the woman's head and pushed the buzzer, though it was distracting and I felt I lost some of the intensity I'd been building up.

During the session I noticed that the volunteer pushed her own button several times. Occasionally Dr. Peper announced over the intercom that my brain waves were changing, and I would concentrate harder on maintaining a steady peak state. Dr. Peper ran several trials, with rest periods in between. It had gone well.

After the test was over, Dr. Peper scanned the chart recorder's printed output and compared the volunteer's chart with mine. At several points our brain-wave patterns were strikingly synchronized, he told us. It also appeared that when I pressed the buzzer to indicate that I was in my most concentrated healing state, the EEG recorded alpha waves, those associated with a deep, meditative state. Dr. Peper was excited about these preliminary findings and suggested to Jim and Roger that I come back the following week for more replications. The repetition was boring, but I understood the necessity—after all, this was science, and testing had to be repeated over and over and over again.

Next we were due at the Institute of Medical Sciences, where we joined Dr. Jerry Jampolsky and Judy Skutch. As we were about to enter this impressive research center, Jerry explained to me that the research director, Dr. Vickers, had requested that there be no unnecessary observers. This was odd—it was the first time that our whole group would not be allowed into an experiment. Rochelle provided important feedback for me—she would watch the processes of different tests, and then we would be able to discuss various aspects and compare notes. We protested, but we followed the rules set for us. No one was pleased to be excluded from this upcoming experiment, but Judy, Rochelle, and Jim finally took off to tour the city, while Jerry, Roger, and I went into the Institute.

When the three of us entered Dr. Vickers's office, he greeted us with a pronounced lack of warmth and enthusiasm. He briskly led us to the lab that had been set aside for our use, pointed to a Plexiglas cage containing the experimental subject—a giant laboratory rat—and introduced us to two lab technicians before making a hasty exit.

By now I was growing accustomed to such treatment from certain scientists, and Vickers's lack of interest didn't bother me a bit. Curious, I walked over to the see-through cage and looked inside at the huge white rat with black spots and a long, skinny tail. It was gross. I had known in advance that I would be working with a rat, but somehow I hadn't expected it to look so repulsive. I recoiled at the sight. I guess I imagined a cute little hamster.

Anxiously I said, "Jerry, I'm not sure I'm going to be able to do this."

I tried to explain that my previous experience with rats had been in the music store, where foot-long rats that lurked in the basement sometimes ventured upstairs and scared the hell out of everybody. I tried to squelch my distaste and sense of foreboding, but I was worried. It had always seemed to me that I needed to have positive thoughts—loving thoughts—toward the subjects I tried to heal. I'd worked before on some friends' cats and dogs—but no rats!

Jerry tried to relieve my distress by distracting me: talking to me and outlining the object of the experiment. I was to try, by means of my energy, to lower the blood pressure of this rat, one of a strain that, otherwise healthy, had been bred specifically for hypertension. The rat's blood pressure and pulse rate would be continually monitored and recorded.

As Jerry checked my own blood pressure before the experiment, I again stressed my trepidation. I knew I couldn't back out of the test, but I wanted to be sure the researchers knew that I doubted my ability to succeed with a subject that generated such repugnant feelings. If they understood that, I was willing to try.

Before the test began, Jerry and Roger were shown into another room. I asked the two technicians if I could be given feedback during the experiment—I wanted to be informed if I was in fact affecting the rodent's blood pressure. During the earlier experiments at SRI with Dr. Peper, I had found that when Peper reported changes in my brain-wave pattern over the intercom, the information somehow enabled me to raise my energy level higher still. If Peper's feedback indicated no change of pattern, I would work harder to produce a larger energy output.

An oscilloscope, a device with a screen on which the rat's pulse rate could be monitored visually, was put within my view. The rat's normal pulse rate was already displayed as wavy horizontal lines. A declining pulse rate would accompany a drop in blood pressure.

When I got the go-ahead from one of the two scientists in the lab with me, I began to concentrate, placing my hands several inches above the plastic see-through enclosure and closing my eyes, for I was truly repulsed by the rat. But no matter how I tried, I could not seem to muster up any love for the creature. I didn't feel that I could open up to the "patient" and make a good connection. For twenty minutes I tried to lower the rat's blood pressure, but each time I glanced at the oscilloscope, the pattern was unchanged. Again, I shut my eyes.

Suddenly, one scientist murmured, "The pulse rate is going down."

I turned to observe the screen again—all eyes were glued to it now—and saw the lines descending. But the technicians were so intent on watching the screen that, without realizing it, they turned the oscilloscope out of my view.

I began to concentrate even more diligently on lowering the rodent's blood pressure. When I asked for someone to tell me whether the rat's pulse rate was still dropping, no one answered. I worked for another ten minutes in the suddenly silent room, then stopped.

Something was wrong, a bit off, but I couldn't put my finger on it. I was ushered into a different room, where Jerry came in and rechecked my own blood pressure, which was normal. He told me to stay there, and left. I was alone for a long time. When he finally returned with Roger and the technicians, their faces bore a mixture of excitement and captivation that I couldn't interpret.

Then Dr. Vickers came in, flanked by six more scientists. Unexpectedly friendly, Dr. Vickers put his arm around my shoulders and asked for my subjective impression of the experiment. I told him that I hadn't been able to shake my loathing for the rat and that after about twenty minutes I had felt something begin to happen, but that I wasn't sure what.

Dr. Vickers then asked me what kind of animals I did like. I probably shouldn't work with rats, he said, in a tone that implied a joke—maybe rabbits would be better. Did I like rabbits? I could not figure out the point of all this banter.

Finally, Jerry interrupted: "Dr. Vickers, don't you think we should tell him?"

And Vickers, still smiling, sat down and told me the results of the test.

"Dean," he said, "the rat you worked on is dead." I felt my heart leap right into my throat.

"Approximately twenty minutes after you began to work on the rat, it died," Vickers went on. "Its blood pressure was so low that its heart stopped."

I was very upset. I could see how intrigued the researchers were, but my own reaction was remorse. If only they had given me the feedback on the rat's blood pressure, as I had asked, I would have stopped working sooner. I had not wanted to kill the poor rat. I felt tired, confused, and disgusted.

As we further discussed the results, I began to understand its implications. It was a little harrowing to think that I could have brought on the rat's death. But the new scientific side of me was also intrigued to think that my fear and loathing of the rat might have led to its demise.

My energy, I supposed, must coordinate with my attitude. I reassured myself, remembering that though I hadn't always personally liked the people I'd treated, I'd always felt a loving connection during healing sessions. And no one ever had experienced a bad side-effect from my treatments.

A postmortem examination would be conducted to see if the exact cause of the rat's death could be determined, the scientists told me. The statistical odds of sudden death in that breed of rat under such experimental conditions would be determined.

When Roger and I returned to Dakin Labs to pick up Rochelle and Judy, they and the Dakin staff were enthralled by our account of the rat experiment. But I was thoroughly drained by the unsettling events of the day.

Rochelle and I slept late the following morning—I always needed a solid nine or ten hours of sleep to feel rested. Luckily we had the day to ourselves until after dinner. We ordered room service and sat in the room all day, discussing the rat experiment. In the evening, several representatives from the government research complex Lawrence Livermore Laboratory met with us and Judy at our hotel. The scientists wanted to discuss the upcoming work with cancer cells.

The researchers quickly explained the point of the scheduled experiment: They wanted to see if I could affect a culture of cancer cells in test tubes. I was gratified that they had brought a film of the microscopic cells, enlarged several thousand times, so that I could see what I would be dealing with. It was *the* most aggressive cancer cell ever known to science—HeLa, named for Henrietta Lacks, a young woman who had died of cervical cancer in 1951. The vicious cancer had quickly run rampant through her body, and when she died, some of her cancerous tissue was removed and grown in cell cultures. This disease, which had become man's worst plight, had been preserved and nurtured so that scientists could conduct experiments to understand it and to see what could destroy it. Medical researchers around the world utilized the infamous HeLa cells in the search for a cancer cure.

We watched the film of the squirmy, oval cells taken as they were about to multiply—approximately every twenty-four hours, each cell splits into two separate cells. "Aggressive" was an understatement! The scientists were looking for any change at all—the breakdown of the adhesive culture, a speeding up or slowing down of reproduction—in the cells or their activity. I was suddenly frightened by the idea of working so closely and directly with these virulent cancer cells, housed only in thin plastic tubes, and I asked about the chance of the disease being transmitted to me. I was told it was highly unlikely, but I did not feel reassured.

I was to begin work on the cells on Monday. The Livermore scientists told me that if I detected any hostility from any of the other researchers at the lab, I should ignore it. It had been very difficult to arrange my visit to Lawrence Livermore, where most researchers were avidly opposed to parapsychology research. *What else is new?* I thought.

The next day, Friday, as Rochelle and I were leaving our hotel room to go to Dakin Labs, we got a call from Dr. Jampolsky about the rat experiment. The autopsy of the dead animal had provided absolutely no explanation for its death. There had been no cerebral hemorrhage, no seizure—the rat's heart had simply stopped. Dr. Vickers also had conducted a quantitative and qualitative statistical analysis, in which he determined that no other rodent had ever died in such a way in a Plexiglas cage. Russell Targ, with whom I'd also worked at SRI, published a book in 1984, *Mind Race,* in which he included this experiment.

That afternoon, Jim Hickman brought us to a room, sat me down, and handed me what looked like a bottle of water. It was actually saline solution, and he wanted me to concentrate on fusing my energy into it. The mixture would then be used to water rye seeds, and their rate of growth would be monitored. A plant watered with a salt solution would be expected to be sickly, and the scientists wanted to see if I could overcome the negative effect of the saline solution by energizing the emulsion.

I suddenly realized that Roger wasn't around, and I asked Jim where he was. Roger would not witness the treatment of the solution, Jim said. In the second part of the experiment, Roger would water the seeds—some with the mixture I treated, and the others with a solution I didn't work on, meant to be the control. It was a blind experiment, meaning Roger would not know which bottle was which.

I felt rather silly treating the saline. Actually, I would have preferred to work directly with the plants or seeds, for it seemed a lot easier to "love" them. I proceeded to pour my energy into the sealed solution.

(It would be two months after I left California before I learned the results of the plant-growth trials. Then I was notified that I had significantly altered the growth of the plants. Those watered with the unhealthy mixture I had treated had grown more slowly than those in the control group, but they had been just as healthy—possibly indicating a "fountain of youth" effect.)

After I finished treating the salted water, Rochelle and I were escorted to the chilly basement, where there was Kirlian photography equipment designed by Henry Dakin. Roger showed us examples of Kirlian photographs that displayed beautifully colored flares emanating from different fingertips.

Test photos of my hands would be taken when I indicated that I was in my healing state, Jim said, and control photos would be taken when

I was not. I was worried that I would have to break my concentration in order to signal Jim, just as I'd had to disrupt my focus to ring the buzzer in Dr. Peper's brain-wave experiments. We worked out the best system we could: Jim would sit next to me, and when I felt at my peak, I would press my knee against his, and he would take a picture. I found it was still distracting.

After several tests, Roger developed the film, and he and Jim said they detected some interesting flares emerging from my hands but that they would have to analyze them further. Science was not a quick-process system—everything took time and repetition. Knowing that some early experiments involving Kirlian photography and healers had not been successfully replicated under stricter controls, I asked if Jim and Roger believed that the flares revealed by Kirlian photography really represented energy emanating from the body. I wasn't surprised when they said they could not be sure. Because so many factors—dirt on the fingers, static electricity, varied pressure on the film plate, changing temperature—could affect the patterns shown in the pictures, they could not make any conclusive statements about the phenomenon except that someday it might be a very useful tool. I myself feel that there are too many variables that can cloud the results.

At the conclusion of the Kirlian trial, Jim and Roger automatically ushered me to the next room, which held the machinery for what they considered to be one of the major parts of the study. On the left side of the large room was a huge, see-through structure of wire mesh, called a Faraday cage. Easily big enough to accommodate fifteen standing adults, the enclosure was designed so experiments could be conducted in a location free of radio waves or magnetic fields—the cage minimized the effects of interference from power lines and radio stations. The purpose of this experiment was to determine if I could produce changes in the electrostatic field within the cage using my own energy.

During the experiment I would sit inside the Faraday cage with my hands resting palms upward on a lapboard. A square metal box would generate an electrostatic field inside the cage in the area above my hands.

The generator was connected by cable to an oscilloscope linked to a chart recorder and a tone feedback system, all located outside the cage. If there were any disturbances in the electrostatic field inside the cage, the steady monotone of the feedback system would change pitch and the chart recorder would indicate the degree to which the field was affected.

All of the equipment inside the cage was so sensitive that movement of any kind could invalidate the tests. Video cameras would be trained on me to assure that I remained perfectly still. Before the test began, my pockets were carefully checked for metal, and then I was instructed to take my seat inside the cage, remove my shoes, roll up my pants legs, and rest my hands on the lapboard. Next I was asked to move my hands in the vicinity of the metal box, while the movement was noted on the chart recorder as an "artifact." In turn, I was told to move my head, my legs, and my toes, and to breathe deeply, so that during the experiment, if any movement was recorded in the cage, the record could be compared with the body artifacts already transcribed. They seemed to be prudent in their precautions—good! I didn't want to hear any bullshit later about lack of controls.

Finally everything was in order. Jim, Roger, and an assistant in charge of the video cameras explained that I was to have sixteen trials. Each trial would be composed of three parts: for forty-five seconds of "experiment" I was to concentrate on affecting the field with my own energy; for forty-five seconds of "control" I was not to affect the field; and for fifteen seconds I was to rest. They would not say in advance which part of the trial they would call for. Jim would randomly say, for example, "Forty-five seconds—experiment," and, as quickly as I could, I would begin to generate energy in an attempt to disturb the electrostatic field being produced inside the cage.

I was intrigued—this was going to be fun! I knew I had the control over my energy that they were searching for and could turn "on" for the experimental period and "off" for the control and rest periods. Indeed, once we began, each time I was given the command for "experiment," I would visualize energy particles rising from my hands toward the metal box, and the feedback tone would instantly change pitch. The tone changed so dramatically that soon the room sounded like a new rock and roll song was being composed just for us.

I remember watching Rochelle standing with Jim and Roger, all of them transfixed to the oscilloscope and chart recorder. Apparently, at times the readings or disturbances went so high that Roger had to turn down the dials to accept the unexpected sky-scraping signals. Each time I concentrated and the field showed changes, Roger would yell, "Yeah! Yeah!" with enormous enthusiasm, urging me on. Then he'd check with the camera person to be certain that I hadn't moved. I had not.

When we left for the weekend, I was tired but content. Throughout the two days off I tried not to think about the tests and have some fun, see a movie—but my thoughts kept drifting back to Monday and my upcoming fight with HeLa. Exposure to these cancer cells in test tubes was still alarming to me because I still was not convinced that the cells were not contagious. After all, the scientists said they hadn't yet discovered what made these hostile and destructive cells "tick." This certainly added to my discomfort. I no longer feared contagion working with people with cancer, but these cells were extremely volatile and still an unknown entity. This is what scared me most.

But after all this buildup, come Monday the Livermore staff was still designing the HeLa experiment, and work was postponed till Friday.

Being disappointed wasn't going to change the adjustment in the schedule, so for the next three days I repeated the Faraday cage experiment at Dakin Labs, with the same tight controls. I affected the field significantly during every trial, each and every day. The experiments were going so well that the atmosphere was almost giddy with comaraderie—Jim and Roger would cheer me on, and their constant feedback really helped me perform at my best.

I participated also in some different brain-wave explorations. A researcher at the Langley Porter Medical Center, Dr. Joe Kamiya—the "father" of biofeedback—was testing for possible correlations of the brain waves of healer and healee, and came up with findings similar to those of Dr. Peper at SRI. There were moments of synchronicity, and my brain waves during healing exhibited a very deep alpha state.

Feeling very confident that evening, Dr. Jampolsky had me try something different during one of the long waiting periods. He had ten cards, each with one of five colors on it, so there were two cards per color. He shuffled the cards and was going to "send" the color he was looking at to me. I was to "receive" and tell him what color he was looking at. I was so jazzed that the moment he glanced at the first one—blue—I immediately rattled off nine more colors. Jampolsky wrote quickly to keep up with me, then checked the cards. He found they corresponded exactly in the order I'd said. He was captivated and dumbfounded with my uncanny accuracy. We had a good laugh.

Dr. Peper also did more EEG recordings, and once again his findings were "intriguing," he said. He wanted to arrange for a full week of testing in the near future. There seemed to be a consistent pattern emerging. He eventually published a book on the subject, using the information already gleaned from our prior work.

Before I knew it, it was Friday, time to face the HeLa cancer cells. I was so exhilarated from the successes I'd already enjoyed during the trip that the HeLa experiment seemed like a bonus. I was almost casual about it. I had finally convinced myself that I could hold the flask of cancer cells without contracting the fatal disease. (My paranoia was not unfounded: It is now a known fact that laboratory workers *are* at a higher risk of catching all sorts of viruses through test-tube handling.)

When Rochelle and I arrived at Livermore Lab, we were subjected to elaborate security checks and given a pass to wear at all times. I was dressed in lightweight cotton clothes, and I had brought along a short-sleeve T-shirt to change into, for I would be working in the "sweatbox"—a small incubator room where the temperature was maintained at 98.6°F and there was only a narrow walkway between two walls that held countless flasks of cancer cells.

The investigator in charge of the experiment, Richard, brought in a "double-eyed" microscope that would permit us to observe simultaneously the malignant cells before and after the trial. Richard pointed to another flask of cells on a shelf and explained that it was the control and would not be touched by me or anybody. He then departed for a meeting, leaving an assistant to monitor the experiment while I concentrated for a half hour on affecting the cells.

To my disappointment, I felt absolutely nothing happen.

We took a lunch break, and I began working again. After about twenty minutes of deep concentration, I began to feel an unmistakable change—a repulsion between my hands and the flask. It was remarkable—it felt as though the cancer cells were resisting me! Then, suddenly, I felt the struggle collapse, as if some of the cells had stopped pushing against me . . . as if they had surrendered.

Tremendously excited, I motioned to the assistant and asked her to check the cells. She became very animated, for there did seem to be a lot of cells floating on top of the solution—many more than before I began to work on them! As the minutes passed, more "floaters," or dead cells, surfaced. The cells were breaking up! I was ecstatic—I knew it! I felt the exact moment it had happened!

When Richard returned from his meeting, he also examined the cells. He and his assistant went into separate rooms to write up their visual observations, then compared them. The reports were quite similar. Richard was obviously shaken.

We were joined by another scientist. He too observed the cells, but his response was that if you shook the flasks, you could get the same result. The assistant immediately took one of the control flasks and shook it vigorously, but the cells remained unaffected. No additional cells died and floated to the top. What was wrong with this guy? If cancer cells could be killed so simply by shaking them, then cancer wouldn't even be around anymore! There would have been a cure decades ago. This guy was ludicrous, but typical.

For yet another opinion, Richard called in a biologist, who seemed very reluctant even to get involved with what we were doing. He looked into the experimental and control flasks and reported emphatically that he saw no difference between them. This bothered Richard, for he and his assistant both had noted a definite difference between the flask I had worked on and the control.

Our group was growing in size as we all paraded through the center into another lab, where Richard put the cells through a Coulter counter, a machine that could count the number of floating cells in a sample. The number of floaters in the control was approximately 530; the number in the flask I had worked on was approximately 1,200—more than twice as many as in the control flask. The biologist, who was still with us, was taken aback and he said he'd like to run the test himself. He did, and the results were the same.

I felt sensational! I had caused cancer cells to break apart under scientifically controlled conditions! No one in the lab ever had seen such a thing happen before, especially from a laying-on-of-hands healer. Now *this* was the research and authentication I had dreamed of!

In addition, the information about my abilities revealed by these experiments pointed to the possible existence of a healing mechanism. The Faraday cage experiments had shown that I could alter an electrostatic field, and an informal test with a magnetometer showed that I had affected a magnetic field. Thus, perhaps I had been able to affect the HeLa cells by altering the electromagnetic force field that surrounds all cells, and that a similar model was at work in my healing of people.

While acknowledging that I had affected the cell cultures, Richard cautioned me not to get carried away. Why not? I wondered. Was he embarrassed of his findings—that a psychic healer had killed cancer cells in test tubes? But his own wonderment was eventually evident, and he proved his dedication to the truth as he started planning a larger-scale series of tests for July. I asked him for a written report, and he said he would mail me one. My growing collection of documentation gave me a tremendous sense of accomplishment.

At thirty thousand feet above sea level and winging our way back to New York, I couldn't help reviewing what had occurred on this eventful and fortuitous two-week research trip. I could not stop thinking also about the repercussions of these amazing studies and how the information would affect the issues and theories on which scientists have based their research. What could this mean for cancer research? What about the contradictions to Newton's laws of gravity? How would this relate to Einstein's theory of relativity?

Killing cancer cells in vitro wasn't the only challenge I had met head-on. There was also my brain-wave tests showing correlations between the patient and me during deep relaxed intervals, the obvious psychokinetic control I was able to display with electrostatic fields in the Faraday cage, and the unfortunate yet spectacular PK effect I had with the rat.

(I was even more gratified a year later, when a report on the healing experiments conducted under the direction of Dakin Labs was submitted as a research brief to the Parapsychology Association for its conference in Utrecht, Holland. Many of my studies were presented, and the reporter who wrote the *Village Voice* article about me told me that he was sitting right next to Dr. Larry LeShan at the conference. While my experiment results were being introduced, LeShan looked very uncomfortable said the reporter. Perhaps LeShan now knew he had called the wrong shot with me. I felt vindicated.)

Still it was difficult for me to comprehend what I had accomplished—I had actually conquered my own doubts and trepidations and had been more successful than the scientists and doctors or even I ever had imagined. I knew it was time for me to establish more of a working relationship with the traditional medical establishment. In my initial experiences, there were only six doctors who were open-minded enough to refer their patients to me. If psychic healing and self-help techniques were to gain widespread credibility, then many more doctors would have to be open to these new avenues of alternative medicine.

11

The Pursuit *of* Credibility: *Documentation and the Medical Establishment*

THE MEDIA CONTINUED TO SEDUCE ME AND REFUSED to allow me out of their enticing widespread grip. In 1975 alone, I appeared on ten radio shows, eight major national television shows, and participated in German, Italian, and American television documentaries on the paranormal. There were also interviews with twenty more newspaper and magazine articles from the United States and around the world. I used the publicity to my advantage and found it an enormously powerful way to spread the message that there are alternatives to consider that work, particularly with problems deemed "hopeless." I felt like I had been handed the torch to proudly lead the way toward respectability and the demystification of laying-on-of-hands energy healing.

The opportunities to present my points of view were difficult to pass up. In fact, in the early years, I had accepted every invitation. I had allowed myself to be extremely accessible, and no magazine, newspaper, or show, known to me or not, had been refused an interview. But now I was much more selective. The question-and-answer sessions usually went well, and I would offer to demonstrate my healing technique, which was always eagerly accepted. I was as passionate in my presentations as I was about every undertaking in my life. And at first it was exciting and novel, but as with anything you have too much of, it grew old.

Of course, there were some original and refreshing interviewers and shows that had presented doctors to speak either in opposition or in support of laying-on-of-hands healing. At this time there still were not enough medical doctors acknowledging the potential of energy healing. I was determined to change that. I found it rewarding to debate these learned professionals, and usually won their respect and interest. And through my demonstrations, some dubious doctor's own pain would go away, or the show's producer's stiff neck was better in moments. There were no doubts about what they felt, for my vibrating hands and the results spoke for themselves. It was reassuring for me to know that I could so easily exhibit my healing technique.

I loved the highly charged atmosphere of a television studio, and found the live audiences very stimulating. I was unshakable in my convictions, and my enthusiasm was usually contagious. Many of these doctors were so unexpectedly impressed with my medical knowledge, research, and positive results that they too soon referred a number of their own patients to me.

My appearance on the network television show *Geraldo Rivera's Goodnight America* in June 1975 was quite a spectacle. A traditional medical doctor was asked to participate in the program to give it "balance." I met him briefly in the "green room," the waiting area designated for the guests, where we had drinks and Rochelle and I conversed with Peter Benchly and Roy Scheider, who were scheduled to be on the segment prior to mine, promoting their new film *Jaws.*

On the show, while giving his report about my work, Geraldo Rivera stated that six ABC staff members had witnessed my performing blatant psychokinesis. When it was time for me to demonstrate my healing art, a much safer undertaking than psychokinesis, Rivera selected his personal secretary, who had back pain, as my subject. Right on camera, as I worked with her, Rivera's secretary said she felt great relief. Rivera, uneasy, turned to the doctor for his opinion. The doctor's candid response was that from what he had just seen, psychic healing seemed to work. Rivera was speechless, but the doctor was impressed enough to refer a patient to me after the taping. This reaction was becoming commonplace. The show also included a segment of the video of me in the lab affecting an electrostatic field. It all went wonderfully.

I was learning to live and appreciate each day more fully, for in life you never know what the next day will bring. A few months later, in August 1975, a tabloid reported on the secretive HeLa cancer cell experiments in which I had participated at Lawrence Livermore Lab. Word of the sensational experiment already had circulated widely throughout the parapsychology community and was mentioned briefly at various conferences and lectures around the country.

The article, when it appeared, was entirely accurate, but it was badly timed. People at Livermore still were sensitive about the publicity that had followed other controversial experiments performed there. For a government-funded research institute affiliated with the Atomic Energy Commission and the University of California to receive publicity about its work with psychics was not good, as far as the director of publicity at the lab was concerned.

The man who had been responsible for getting me into Livermore called me, frantic. He had been reprimanded and was now *forbidden* from doing any more psychic research at the lab. That meant that I would not be given the opportunity to repeat the HeLa cancer cell experiment there. He told me that even if I were to go to Livermore and levitate all the desks in the complex, the lab still would not want to have anything to do with psychic research. He was concerned about his job and passionately urged me to burn any papers given to me by the lab, especially my copy of an interdepartmental memo that confirmed the results of my experiments with the cancer cultures.

This was a bitter blow. Of course, putting a lit match to those papers was out of the question! Indeed, I became only more intent on repeating the experiment at another prominent laboratory. How ironic it would seem later when I found out that Livermore's major research effort at the time was the development of a neutron bomb. I guess they preferred to research killing people rather than killing cancer!

•

It was December 6, 1975, when Rochelle and I sat in a white limousine, nervously waiting for the most important moment of our lives. After all these years of anticipation and preparation, the time had finally arrived. Today, everything else in our lives took a backseat.

We stepped out into the cold pelting rain, and Rochelle's gorgeous off-white beaded wedding gown and headdress, and my own hunter-green tuxedo, were getting soaked. But we could not have cared less, because after seven years of knowing and loving each other, we were finally getting married.

I felt fortunate that Rochelle and I knew each other before I became a healer and embarked on this odyssey. She loved me for myself and not because I have these paranormal gifts. Rochelle automatically tried to create a normal environment in an abnormal life.

She keeps me grounded and my ego humbled, calms me when things get hairy, and consoles me when I'm in despair. She sets up our work schedule, puts in the same hours as I do, and takes care of all the normal things of life. Surrounding me in a loving and secure aura, Rochelle has helped me to create miracles. I am certain we were destined to be together.

More than one hundred fifty people came to help celebrate our long-awaited special moment. Some of them were patients who could not walk before seeing me, and were now dancing at my wedding.

•

It was now October 11, 1976, and I had accepted an invitation from a news television station in New York to come to their studio and demonstrate on the air. One of their employees, who had a constantly painful back resulting from a severe kidney condition that the doctors couldn't help, was selected as my patient. To my dismay, I was assigned the most obnoxious reporter I had ever encountered.

The reporter's hostility to Rochelle, me, and the subject matter was immediately made evident upon our arrival at the studio. He had an arrogant attitude toward the field and us, and even had an argument with Rochelle regarding his interpretation of the patient's condition. Of course, we should have just left the studio, but it was too late.

After successfully treating and relieving the employee of his pain, on film, I felt this reporter could not do anything to hurt me or the field. After all, I had accomplished what had been asked of me—I had helped their choice of patient while demonstrating my technique.

Were we in for a shock! That afternoon, we sat in our New York office and watched the taped show on television. Rochelle and I were horrified. The reporter had added a voice-over editorial comment after my successful demonstration: "But because of Kraft's prior dealings in the occult, a shadow of doubt hangs over the credibility of psychic healing."

It was remarkable that this man's arrogant disbelief was being used to discredit what the film actually had captured. Rochelle felt awful, for she believed she was responsible for this nightmare—she was the one who had insisted that he report accurately, but I knew there was much more to it than that.

I immediately called the director of the station and threatened to file a lawsuit based on defamation of character and reporting an outright lie. He immediately got his reporter on the line and asked him point blank, with Rochelle and me listening in, "What is your source of information for that voice-over comment you added on to the news piece?"

After the reporter stammered a bit, it came out—because of the *Voice* article discussing the unusual car-door lock episode, he had interpreted this event (incorrectly) as "occult" and therefore to be discounted. He was fired on the spot. When we all hung up, Rochelle and I felt so badly about the outcome that I called back and tried to discourage the director from taking the actions he had, and actually tried to get the reporter reinstated. But the station director refused.

I became obsessed with carefully documenting and proving my abilities. I knew the credibility I sought for my healing work lay in the hands of the doctors, the ultimate and most prestigious group to oversee and certify my gifts. I still strongly believed in the validity of medical science. After all, their diagnostic procedures had provided me with clinical information, which assisted me in helping people.

I always encouraged my patients to continue with their physicians' courses of care and insisted they take their prescribed medications and treatments. My stand of not being an alternative, but rather an adjunct, to doctors helped bridge my relationships and respect with the medical community.

This public position put me in demand to lecture at hospitals, medical centers, colleges, as well as the Women's House of Detention on Riker's Island in New York. One presentation in particular was a Grand Rounds meeting at Albert Einstein College of Medicine's Lincoln Hospital in the Bronx, which was arranged by Dr. David Laskowitz, a prominent psychologist at the hospital, who had an interest in parapsychology and had heard me speak on a radio program.

Dr. Laskowitz's fascination with that program led him to my second seminar, held at the Hilton Hotel in New York City, where I taught more than two hundred people how to help themselves and others through the laying on of hands. After the full-day program, Laskowitz approached me about his chronic back problem. He said his back felt much better after utilizing the self-healing exercises I'd taught that afternoon, but asked if he could come in to see me to experience my touch directly. We had two sessions together, and his problem was gone. Thus he was prompted to recommend some of his own patients to me, and they, too, were benefited. Dr. Laskowitz was now ready to share his find with his peers at the Grand Rounds.

I was honored to give the monthly address, which was intended to keep hospital doctors up-to-date on new research and general medical information and was usually delivered by a physician. As Dr. Laskowitz guided me into the large lecture room, my stomach was already dealing with a huge invasion of butterflies. Even though I had spoken publicly many times before, this was different, for everyone attending this lecture was a medical doctor trained in traditional Western medicine. I believed this would be the ultimate acid test—to see if these physicians would be able to put aside their scientific logic and medical doctrine, which basically taught them that what I'd been doing all these years did not exist. I was hoping they at least would be open-minded to the possibilities that the laying on of hands has a real positive effect in improving the health and hopes of others.

I knew it would be a challenge for me to win over this reputable and primarily skeptical audience. But I was prepared to do some demonstrations, for, in past lectures, these displays hit the mark when audience members came to me with pain and walked away without it. Afterward, it would be difficult for them to remain skeptical.

The lecture room was full, and there seemed to be fifty or sixty doctors in attendance. I was told it was a packed house—word had spread that today's Grand Round meeting was going to be unusual. As I sat in the front row reviewing my notes on index cards, Dr. Laskowitz stood at the podium and introduced me. He began by relaying his experience at the seminar and how I'd helped him and some of his patients. He felt there was "something there" and medical science needed to take a closer, objective look at the usefulness of this complementary therapy. Dr. Laskowitz even said that since learning my laying-on-of-hands techniques, he himself had helped two patients of his own with arthritis. Then he discussed the positive value of doctors' learning my techniques and even suggested it be taught in medical schools.

The butterflies in my stomach flew away as soon as I spoke my first words: "It is a real privilege to be given this podium and to be the first laying-on-of-hands healer to speak before you, and to be allowed to share my ideas and research with such an esteemed audience. I can only hope your minds will open to the importance and need for a laying-on-of-hands healer to be in every hospital. I would also like to discuss the unfortunate void in the 'hope' department in the medical establishment and how essential even a little touch of hope is for many patients that are in terminal situations. Hope fuels the will to live. . . ." And I was on my way, barely glancing at my notes.

Time seemed to speed by as I got into communicating with the interested audience. I really felt I was making an impact. Then I discussed the possible applications that the doctors themselves could integrate into their own specialties and practices. I spoke of the need to utilize more placebos and incorporate this harmless treatment into the medical system when all other conventional medical avenues fail.

In addition, I mentioned the importance of a better working relationship between the energy healer and the medical doctor to properly observe and document the patient's results as well as the treatment's efficacy. And, last but not least, I stressed the need for more research into energy healing and other similar alternative therapies.

Then I asked for volunteers who had pain at that moment, and twenty hands must have shot up into the air. I had two doctors join me at the podium and sat them on straight-backed chairs.

The gray-templed male physician was in his mid-fifties and had a lower-back problem, and the other doctor, a woman in her early forties, had a migraine headache in full bloom—I could sense the pain from her eyes. Both seemed doubtful that I would be able to alleviate their pain right away, and that only fueled my desire to help them and raised my energy level even higher.

After instructing them to close their eyes and focus on their breathing, I began to work on the subject who had lower-back pain. I placed my left hand two inches from his forehead, and my right hand about an inch from his back, and within two minutes he remarked about feeling waves of heat going into him.

He was somewhat off-balance, and asked, "Are you touching me?" His face went beet red when some of his compatriots in the audience smiled and shook their heads—no, I was not.

I continued holding that position for a couple of minutes more, and then turned to the migraine case. I heard a murmuring of voices through the room and knew I had their attention and fascination. I placed my left hand a couple inches away from her forehead, my right hand gently at the back of her head, and proceeded to generate energy.

Within moments she exclaimed, "His hands are hot as irons! And I'm feeling this really strange vibration throughout my whole body."

I remained in this position for a couple more minutes, then removed my hands and turned back to the other doctor. I asked him, "How's the pain—is it as severe as when we started?" During normal treatment sessions I never ask, but I do during demonstrations.

The blushing doctor replied, "No, not at all. Honestly it feels about ninety-percent better—I really can't believe it!" A swell of excited voices swept through the room.

Then I asked the migraine case how she was doing. She too was red-faced, and exclaimed, "It's gone—my migraine is gone! That was unbelievable! How did you do that?"

The two doctors I'd worked on started addressing each other, comparing notes on what they felt, and many people in the audience began shouting out questions.

"One at a time," I yelled above the buzz. "Be patient; I'll get to all of you."

The group was revved up over what they'd just witnessed. They asked the standard *How?, When?,* and *Why?,* and my responses were as rapid-fire as their inquiries. I ended up staying an hour and a half longer than expected in order to answer all their queries. I was satisfied: The meeting had gone very well, even better than I had hoped.

Then Dr. Seymour Grossman, a psychiatrist in New York City and a member of the President's Board of Psychiatry, became another public supporter of my alternative procedure. Interestingly enough, Grossman had heard of me through one of his own patients who was under his care for chronic depression, whom I had helped with a bad back. Dr. Grossman said that since seeing me, the patient was progressing more quickly toward better mental health.

The doctor wanted to know if I was interested in working my "unique skills," as he called them, on a highly unusual case of his—a catatonic patient. I was intrigued with this new situation and quickly looked up "catatonic" in my medical dictionary. It is a condition in which a person, commonly schizophrenic, becomes physically rigid, sometimes unconscious, but more often violent. This would certainly be a challenge of notable proportions! I approached it with my natural fervor. Dr. Grossman would observe the sessions, and afterward, sometimes over dinner, we would discuss the progress.

The patient, Allan, never said a word, only made some deep guttural sounds and moved around a bit within the confines of his wheelchair while I worked with him. Grossman's interpretation of these actions was that Allan was feeling something different—his movements were considerably more sedate whenever I treated him.

Dr. Grossman seemed quite impressed with these small changes. I, of course, was looking for the big effects, like for Allan to jump out of his chair and begin an intelligent conversation with us, even though he hadn't moved with coordination or spoken in years. My expectations were always aimed toward the moon, and most times I accomplished the task, but not always to my satisfaction. Still, I was pleased with the continuing number of physicians interested in my work.

It was through Dr. Grossman that three-month-old Jennifer Paul was brought to my office by her parents. Jennifer had been born with severe nerve damage and an inner-ear malfunction, and had been pronounced "severely to profoundly deaf" by an otolaryngologist at Long Island Jewish Hospital and by the director of the Lexington School for the Deaf. Though only an infant, she was already enrolled at the school, but the only help they offered was a tiny hearing aid and eventual speech therapy. Jennifer's unfortunate condition was considered incurable.

I asked the young mother to sit on my recliner, with Jennifer on her knees. As I carefully focused my energy on the baby's head and ears for a few minutes, Irwin Paul said that since his daughter's hearing had just been tested at her school—the test had revealed a 70-percent hearing loss—any improvement would be easy to gauge.

A few weeks later, Mr. Paul called with wonderful news. Since my session with Jennifer, she had seemed to be more responsive to his voice and to other sounds, and he had just taken her for retesting. Mr. Paul started to choke up as he told me that the new test indicated a hearing loss of only 30 percent. The Lexington School personnel had been unable to explain this sudden and unexpected improvement. They had simply removed Jennifer's hearing aid and told her astonished father that she could no longer be enrolled in a program for the hearing impaired.

Mr. Paul, a high-school guidance counselor and former science teacher, was what I call an open-minded skeptic. He respected scientific principles but was willing to look beyond their boundaries. He told me candidly that he didn't know whether to attribute Jennifer's improvement to my treatment or to a miraculous coincidence. All he knew for sure was that right after he had brought Jennifer to see me, she had begun to hear, and the doctors didn't know why.

The last time I heard from Jennifer's parents, her hearing had improved until *no deficiency at all* could be detected. I had never worked on an infant before, and I was moved by the idea of restoring the priceless gift of hearing to a tiny baby. I was overjoyed that little Jennifer, expected to grow up deaf, would instead have a normal life, filled with the richness of sound that most of us take for granted. Her life had been changed at its very outset. Certainly, the healings of some of my more mature patients had given me pleasure when the end of illness had enabled them to return to a way of life that had once been full but that seemed in danger of being taken from them forever. But the case of Jennifer Paul also proved incredibly important in my search for corroboration of my healing ability. This three-month-old tot had been declared clinically deaf before I treated her, and now she could hear. Let someone try to take this cure and attribute it to "suggestion"!

Like the situation with Jennifer Paul, the case of Robert Lewin enabled me to secure additional acknowledgment from the world of traditional medicine. Lewin, a thirty-eight-year-old real-estate agent, had visited his ophthalmologist a week before his first session with me. His visual acuity was near normal—in his right eye, but he was severely nearsighted—in his left eye. The doctor also had discovered an old scar with a small hemorrhage above it at the back of his left eye, which was obstructing Robert's vision.

Since doctors at Montefiore Hospital didn't think there was much of a possibility of halting the degeneration of his eyesight, he wanted to give my treatment a chance.

Nine days after our first session, Robert returned to his doctor and was told that the vision in his left eye had improved to 20/200, though there had been no change in the hemorrhage in the rear of the eye. Still, Robert and I were encouraged by that initial improvement, and Robert began coming to me regularly. As time passed he reported that his vision had cleared noticeably. After eight months he returned to his opthalmologist.

This time Robert's good right eye had improved a bit, to 20/25. However the vision in his left eye had increased dramatically, to 20/50, and the bleeding at the back of the eye was gone. At my request, Robert had his doctor write up his findings in a letter confirming these changes. My documentation was growing by leaps and bounds.

I was delighted when Bernard Hanover, M.D., from New York referred Robert Bennet, a middle-aged man with severe back, groin, and thumb-joint pain. After only a few sessions, I received a letter from Dr. Hanover himself, reporting that 75 percent of Robert's groin pain, 50 percent of his back pain, and all of the thumb pain had disappeared after the sessions with me. In addition, he thanked me for seeing his patient.

A young lady with severe scoliosis, a painful curvature of the spine, with accompanied head pain was referred by neurologist Dr. Gabriel Rubin. She had been seen by all the best specialists, but none could offer her relief. After only a few sessions with me, the pain disappeared and the curve in her spine lessened by several degrees. She told Dr. Rubin: "My sessions with Dean were phenomenal, and he was giving off some kind of energy from his hands."

In constant motion, running as fast as I could toward my goals, I was compelled to begin teaching my laying-on-of-hands techniques to medical doctors. It was obvious to me that my earlier talk at Lincoln Hospital had gone well, and Dr. Michael O. Smith, who had attended the Grand Rounds lecture and was the director of the Drug Detoxification Program at Lincoln Hospital, was open to and supportive of my theory that my methods could be taught. His interest prompted me to fine-tune my step-by-step technique so that *others* could follow.

I presented this method to Dr. Smith, a likeable, dark-haired man about my size, and we arranged for my return to the hospital to teach my technique to him and the other doctors in charge of the detox program. Within weeks, I was walking the rough streets of the Bronx to Lincoln Hospital. My new "students" were as eager as I.

First I led the doctors through the process of relaxing their own bodies and minds. Then I instructed them to lightly place their thumbs together on the patient's mid-forehead, forming a "butterfly" with their hands above the eyes. Next, I trained them to visualize a *connection* between themselves and the ill person. This connection would be in the form of the figure-eight lying on its side—the left side being the healer, the right side the patient. I would then have them visualize a white light going from one half of the eight to the other, and back again. By focusing on this image, the doctors could stimulate the patient's own healing mechanism. The process is similar to the way a car battery charges up a weakened one.

Then I told the doctors to concentrate on light and heat, propelled and controlled by their own slow breathing, circling the ill person's body and expanding in width as it passes over afflicted areas. After each cycle around the recipient, the energy should be drawn back to the healer, then sent out again.

I also showed them how to make their patients more receptive using certain physical- and mental-relaxation techniques. Finally, I explained how they could teach their patients self-help visualization exercises.

It was a long, intense day, but at the conclusion, after each doctor had alternately played "healer" and "patient" to practice what he or she had just learned, the doctors were extremely pleased with the session. So was I. Actually, I was delighted with their enthusiasm and willingness to learn and apply my alternative method. Dr. Smith subsequently told the London *Daily Mail* that the detox unit uses my techniques regularly and successfully in lessening the pain, anxiety, and depression that often result from the withdrawal of alcohol and other drugs.

Another good reason for teaching doctors the laying on of hands is that it increases their sensitivity and leads them to giving their patients a little more tender loving care. Many doctors have confirmed that a warm, caring attitude is notably lacking in modern medical practices. It was illuminating for me to see these professionals becoming cognizant of the need for better comforting techniques and a more kindhearted bedside manner.

When evidence of the success of alternative healing was presented to some skeptical physicians, they commonly responded that the healing must be caused by suggestion or placebo. But recent research into the relationship of mind and body has made it impossible for scientists to dismiss lightly the "placebo effect" phenomenon—inert, harmless placebo pills actually do create a physical effect after all. In fact, after a subject is given a placebo or sugar pill, a *physiological* change actually takes place in the brain, which then produces opiatelike substances called endorphins. These brain chemicals are the body's own natural painkillers. Perhaps more powerful than any available medication, they act on specific receptors in the brain and spinal cord, just as morphine and other narcotics do. Additional substances also are produced by the brain in response to the stimulus of a placebo.

If a harmless sugar pill can cause the brain to formulate substances that alleviate pain, a similar model may be at work in the effectiveness of all healing procedures, including Western medicine, hypnosis, acupuncture, chiropractology, homeopathy, and psychic healing. If a person believes he is doing something to help himself, that in itself can act as a healing catalyst.

I have always felt that as long as an alternate healing method cannot harm you, there is no reason for doctors, family, or friends not to look at, study, and try other alternative approaches, especially if traditional routes have been exhausted and the prognosis is poor. There are doctors who argue that it is unethical to raise the hopes of terminally ill patients, but I believe that hope should be the very first thing that is administered—it is the first step in refueling the will to live.

One famous case regarding this very issue occurred in April 1975, when a young woman in her early twenties from New Jersey, Karen Ann Quinlan, was given up as hopeless. Following an evening of, apparently, two gin and tonics and a few Valium pills, she fell into a coma. After months of no improvement in Karen's condition, she was deemed brain-dead. Her family wanted to pull the plug on her life-preserving breathing machine. This created quite a legal stir.

Within a short time, I was contacted by her legal guardian and attorney, Daniel Coburn. He told me that he felt the family had not exhausted all possible avenues of hope and wanted to know if I would like to be involved. I was ready to jump in headfirst. Coburn gathered letters from some of the medical doctors with whom I was working. The documents stated that, based on the fact that I had helped a number of their own hopeless or unresponsive patients, they were in full support of my being given a chance to try to help Karen.

It was an exciting time for me. I held strong views on life-and-death issues and was looking forward to being involved in the case and to my first visit with Karen. I was disappointed when Coburn eventually called to say that even though he was Karen's guardian, he still had to get her parents' approval, and they were resisting any intervention.

I felt sad that Karen was denied my help. Every case is different, but I have come to believe that pulling the plug should be resorted to only when the person involved has given his or her prior consent or instructions in a living will. Regardless if the patient is an adult or a young child, the person should be allowed many months, if not longer, to let the body try to heal from whatever trauma resulted in that deep unconscious state. Alternative therapies definitely should be offered.

I never stopped wondering about these gifts of mine and their baffling and bizarre origins. What were the limits to my abilities? Was there more to discover—other abilities I was not yet aware of? These questions soon were answered in ways I never had expected.

12

Psychic Detective

SINCE CHILDHOOD I HAVE BEEN FASCINATED WITH detective stories. I have spent many a night glued to the television set, watching *Kojak* or *Police Story* reruns. Little did I know that this fascination would eventually lead me to a harrowing experience that had me literally in fear for my life.

From the time I'd heard about Peter Herkos, a well-known Dutch psychic who worked with the police in solving crimes and finding missing people, I was captivated by the idea of an alliance between psychics and the police. I felt that my own direction was healing, but I always wondered where the boundaries of my psychic abilities lay.

When I was first asked to try psychometry and I was able to receive strong feelings about the recently deceased woman whose keys I held, I became aware that my powers might not be exclusive to healing, psychokinesis, and clairvoyance. I felt I was still an untapped source.

My first attempt at psychic detective work had been back in 1974 in my folks' living room, which, at that time, still served as my office. I had received a call from a New Jersey attorney, Peter Cory, who explained that his dilemma was not a health problem. His rebellious sixteen-year-old daughter, Patty, had been missing for three weeks, and though she had run away before, she had never been gone so long without contacting some member of the family. Knowing only too well the dangers that teenage runaways could encounter, Peter Cory asked me to try to help locate his child.

The thought of putting my psychometry ability to another test had been intriguing, and I decided to give it a try. I listened to Mr. Cory's account of some of his daughter's escapades, but I felt I needed more information—perhaps a picture. I had heard that in similar cases, other psychics used pictures to help spark intuitive or extrasensory flashes.

A few days later, I received an envelope containing the most recent picture Mr. Cory had of Patty. She was thin, with long, straight, light-brown hair, and she looked much younger than sixteen. I read Mr. Cory's letter, which restated many of the facts he had told me over the phone, then studied the photo, trying to reach deep within myself for any kind of strong feelings, a mental picture, any connection at all. But I felt nothing.

Then I remembered that when I had first performed psychometry, holding the keys in my hand had definitely set something off inside of me. I contacted Mr. Cory again and asked him to send me a personal item that belonged to Patty.

In two days I received a special-delivery package containing a pair of earrings that Patty often had worn. Sitting at my desk, I carefully placed the earrings in the center of my left palm and immediately felt a quickening of my pulse. I closed my eyes and forced myself to breathe slowly, calming myself so that any psychic impressions could flow freely. The earrings seemed to come alive in my hand.

With my right hand I absently picked up a pen and began to sketch on a white pad. It was completely involuntary—I felt that I was not in control of the pen. I concentrated intently on making a psychic connection with Patty Cory, and an image began to form in my mind. Then I looked down at the paper and saw the picture developing there, like a photographic image emerging on blank paper in a darkroom.

I watched my hand as it began to draw automatically. The light sketch lines turned into a building, a luncheonette on a street corner. The luncheonette had a large white sign, and I could clearly see vivid blue lettering advertising home-cooked meals and a friendly element. My pen continued to move across the paper, and an L-shaped motel appeared just opposite the café. Tension began to build in my body as I felt myself getting closer to an answer. Then another large concrete building appeared. It was a discotheque.

Pulling back, I realized that I had drawn what appeared to be a section of a beach town or resort area. I had depicted a very wide expanse of beach—wider than any I could recall ever having seen at the time—at the right side of the picture. Then the name "Wildwood" flashed like a bolt of lightning across my bewildered mind.

I immediately called Mr. Cory, fumbling so with excitement that I had to dial his phone number three times. He was stunned. Of course, he said, there was a town named Wildwood on the Atlantic coast of New Jersey. This information fit in with the immense beach area that I had seen.

In response, I instructed Mr. Cory to be in Wildwood on Thursday if he wanted to find his daughter. I didn't know why Thursday had come to mind, but I felt it was very important. Mr. Cory said he'd be in Wildwood, accompanied by the local police, as soon as possible. Even though I didn't want to sound pushy, I felt compelled to repeat that he should be there no later than Thursday.

I must not have been emphatic enough, for Peter Cory called me the next weekend and told me that he and the police had gone to Wildwood, but not until Saturday. He hadn't found his daughter. Still, Mr. Cory described the beach town exactly as I had seen it—an L-shaped motel, a disco down the block, a luncheonette on the corner with blue lettering on the sign! Moreover, he had shown Patty's picture to the local people, and she had been positively identified by several employees of the motel and disco. But apparently she had left town on Friday!

I was frustrated, and I supposed I had heard the last of Peter Cory. But about three weeks later he phoned and told me my information had been most helpful after all. He and the police had followed up the leads they had uncovered in Wildwood, and had finally found Patty, in good health, in another nearby resort area. This news had been enormously encouraging, and I was learning more and more to retain confidence in my intuitions.

So when, two years later, the opportunity to play psychic detective and work with the New York Police Department presented itself, I felt ready. In 1976, I got a call from Detective John McGrath of the Brooklyn Robbery Squad, who had been referred by Judy Skutch. (Judy, by that time, was withdrawing from the research end of parapsychology and was devoting her attention into publishing *A Course in Miracles* with her new Foundation for Inner Peace. She told me I had been her inspiration.)

Judy had mentioned to him my fascination with psychic detective work, and he wanted to know if I would like to tackle a robbery case that had the police baffled. I was indeed eager to see if I could help, and I invited the detective to my office.

Later that day, Rochelle escorted two plainclothes detectives into my office. Detective McGrath was a towering, friendly man in his late thirties, with red hair and a thick mustache. He wore a sport jacket, an open-necked shirt, and tan slacks. He introduced his companion, whose cool attitude felt like a sudden chill wind in the room, but I ignored it as McGrath described his own background. The holder of a master's degree in forensic psychology, McGrath had originated a hypnosis program at the police department, taught hypnosis courses at the police academy, and was clearly an innovative thinker in criminal work. He was fascinated by psychics and enthusiastic about using them to help solve difficult cases. Already he had worked with two psychics in the past, and he said their aid had been valuable.

Then McGrath profiled the case at hand. Only a few days before, $500,000 had been stolen from a Hassidic rabbi and his two daughters, who had just withdrawn the money from a Manhattan bank. The police had no solid leads.

I started to relax in my chair, asking the detectives to take notes on anything I said. Excitement was welling up as I suddenly began to see pictures and words forming in my mind. This experience was different from earlier ones—the information was coming so fast. I felt a thick lump developing in my chest as mental images flashed like neon signs.

"The robbers live in Brooklyn, maybe in the Bensonhurst or Bay Ridge sections," I told the policemen, suddenly feeling great confidence in this information.

"One of the perpetrators," I added, self-consciously using what I supposed was police language, "lives on Eighty-sixth Street and Twenty-first Avenue. The money was dropped off near there, around Eighty-sixth Street and Bay Parkway."

I took a breather. The second detective was looking at me skeptically, but Detective McGrath was enthralled, sitting on the edge of his seat and hanging on everything I said. Then another word flashed before me: "Joey." I was sure that one of the robbers was named Joey.

The second detective checked his list of possible suspects, smirking as he told me that there was no Joey there. But he added the name to the list. Then I was exhausted. All the information I had related had seemed to flow easily enough, but now I was drained of strength and energy.

After the detectives left, promising to call if there was any progress in the case, Rochelle came into my office, eager to know the details of their visit. When I recounted what had happened, her only concern was for my safety: What if "Joey" found out that I had put the finger on him? I finally convinced her that wouldn't happen, but I failed to convince myself.

Two weeks after my meeting with McGrath, he called in with great excitement to tell me that the leads I had given him had proven to be exactly right! The stolen money had been dropped off near an ice-cream parlor on Eighty-sixth Street and Bay Parkway in the Bensonhurst–Bay Ridge section of Brooklyn. The police had retrieved some of the money, though part of it was missing. Two suspects had been identified. One of them resided near the ice-cream parlor, at Eighty-sixth Street and Twenty-first Avenue. But he was dead—his body had been found in New Jersey, lying near a car belonging to the second suspect. The dead man's name: Joey.

I was awed by what McGrath told me. These curious abilities of mine were proving to be on the mark much more consistently than I ever had hoped.

Three months later, Detective McGrath called again. The police had just apprehended the second robbery suspect at Kennedy Airport. He was carrying $140,000 of the stolen money. Detective McGrath told me emphatically that he was very impressed by the accuracy of my information, which he said went "beyond luck." Though he had consulted psychics in the past, he said, none had ever been quite as accurate as I. But, he added, police don't really know how to utilize the information they get from psychics who are working with them.

"You're dealing in a time and space frame that the police department doesn't know how to deal with," he told me. "It will take us time to catch up to your abilities and use your information more accurately."

Several months went by, and Detective McGrath contacted me again. This time he asked if I would like to get involved in a mysterious year-old homicide case. The police department had already authorized my immediate involvement. A mixture of vanity and curiosity prompted my instant agreement. I loved to be tested, challenged.

Within days Detective McGrath came to my office with Detective John O'Flaherty, a veteran of the homicide squad, who told me he'd never worked with a psychic before but that he'd been extremely impressed with my work on the robbery. O'Flaherty related the facts of the homicide case: A year earlier, a Brooklyn man in his early forties had started his day as usual, breakfasting with his wife and two children and kissing them good-bye before leaving for work. He was never seen again. The police had discovered his beat-up cream-colored Ford Fairlane parked down by the docks in south Brooklyn. A tremendous amount of the man's blood and brain matter were splattered over the front seat and around the car, and his tortoiseshell-framed glasses, stained with blood and missing one lens, lay inside. But there was no body. After a year the police still hadn't found the corpse and didn't have the vaguest idea who had killed the man.

McGrath pulled out an envelope containing two photographs—one of the murdered man and another of his car—and the man's bloodied eyeglasses. I held the glasses in my hand while I studied the pictures, but I didn't feel any sensations from them. What I did feel was the desire to see, perhaps even sit in, the dead man's car, and I told the detectives so. I was surprised at myself—blood and guts were fascinating, but only on television. Actually, I can be rather squeamish around blood.

My office wasn't far from the victim's home, so Detective McGrath suggested we go there. The man's widow worked near her home and I could get a feel for his neighborhood before sitting in the car. As we left my office, the detectives pointed to a taxi parked across the street—their unmarked vehicle. As I slid into the backseat I couldn't help but think, *Move over, Kojak!*

Our first stop was Bensonhurst, Brooklyn, where the murdered man had lived peacefully with his family. As we slowly cruised the residential street, O'Flaherty pointed out the murdered man's house—one of the row of seven or eight similar houses, red brick, with five steps leading to the front door. McGrath discreetly pointed to a huge, rough-looking man in a long leather jacket who was talking to a shorter, slighter man on the street near the victim's house. The big man was a suspect in the case, McGrath explained, for he'd been reported to have exchanged threats with the victim after a domestic dispute. He was known to get into fights frequently, and he had a criminal record. Viewing the two men on the street, I felt certain that if I could somehow look into the suspect's eyes, I could tell if he was involved in the case.

O'Flaherty turned the corner, stopped the cab, and asked if I had gotten any special feelings about the suspect as we passed him. I told him about my desire to look the man in the eyes. Eager to assist me, O'Flaherty suggested that he and McGrath "cover" me while I approached the man under the ruse of asking for directions.

I could hardly believe what I had gotten myself into, but I watched as the cops took their positions. McGrath remained on the corner near where we had parked, and O'Flaherty jogged briskly around the block to the far corner, beyond the spot where the two men were talking.

After getting a slight nod from McGrath, I slowly made my way down the lengthy street. I tried to appear casual, but I did glance over my shoulder once, to see McGrath lounging against a building, apparently reading a newspaper. Then I looked toward the corner ahead of me, but at first I couldn't see O'Flaherty. I felt a quiver in the pit of my stomach. What the hell was I doing here? I felt some relief when I finally saw O'Flaherty watching me discreetly, his head barely visible. But still I was scared.

I finally drew near the two strangers, and when the man in question noticed me, I quickly walked up to him and asked for some directions, making sure to look directly into his eyes, which were dark brown and piercing.

Immediately I felt great relief, for I sensed that, in this case, the man was innocent. Though certainly no boy scout, he was not the murderer. When our eyes met, my fears dissipated a bit, and I knew I was in no immediate danger. I thanked the man for his help and turned and walked back up the block. My heart was still pounding so hard it almost hurt, but I concentrated on moving slowly and naturally. When I turned the corner, both detectives were waiting for me, eager to hear my impressions of the suspect. I told them that my strong intuition was that the man was not who they were looking for.

Back in the taxi, I already felt headachy and tired, but I ignored my feelings and asked the detectives what our next stop was. They drove down another street in the neighborhood and pointed out a dry-cleaning store, where a pale and drawn-looking middle-aged woman sat, bent over a sewing machine near the window. She was the dead man's widow. McGrath led me into the store and introduced me to the woman. I chatted nonchalantly with her for a few moments, but I didn't get any special feelings about the case from her other than deep sadness.

From the store we drove toward the Brooklyn docks, where the man's car had been found. I wondered whether I could feel anything from the supposed scene of the murder, since it had happened more than a year before. Also, the car might have been transported from another location after the murder was committed.

We parked in the spot where the vehicle had been discovered, and I closed my eyes, trying to clear my mind of thoughts and fears. It wasn't easy, for I was growing weary. Again, I felt nothing significant, so I suggested once more that I actually sit in the car in which the murder had taken place. The car was being held at an old police compound in a housing development in Brooklyn, and we decided to make that our final stop for the day.

We found the Ford parked at the rear of the compound. I looked inside and saw the dark bloodstains and what I imagined to be bits of human tissue. McGrath covered the seat with a big white sheet and, cracking a joke to break the tension, invited me to sit inside. Then he and O'Flaherty went to wait for me in the taxi.

As I lowered my body onto the front seat, I felt the cool autumn wind raise goose bumps on my arms. There was a terrible odor in the car, and it made me queasy. Almost without realizing it, I began to hyperventilate. The pain in my lungs was strong, and the nausea kept rising though I fought to hold it down.

Then a picture—a clear image in vivid color—blazed in my mind. I saw a short, stocky man with a pasty, pock-marked complexion, curly black hair, and a wide hooked nose. I felt my pulse race as I focused on his long, white apron, the kind worn by a butcher. It was covered with dark-red stains. My mind ached.

As though I were watching a slide show, a new image flashed into place. It was a gun—a silver .38 with a mother-of-pearl handle. Part of the butt was broken off.

Then, quite abruptly, I knew that I had received all the impressions I was going to while sitting in the car. I was glad to be finished. I got out, leaving the sheet covering most of the mess, and went to O'Flaherty and McGrath.

I described the images I had received, and when I ended, O'Flaherty's face was drained of all color. Wordlessly he removed a photo I hadn't seen before, a black-and-white Polaroid from his shirt pocket, and handed it to me. There was the same man I had seen—dark curly hair, hooked nose, pitted complexion, and bloodied apron. He was the dead man's brother-in-law, McGrath told me excitedly. He had recently become a suspect because he had expressed excessive concern over his relative's death.

As McGrath drove me to Rochelle's parents' house, where Rochelle was waiting for me, he told me that for some time the police had suspected that the murder was somehow connected with a meat-packing conspiracy. He and O'Flaherty decided they would like me to go with them to a meat-packing plant, where I might obtain further clues as to the location of the dead man's body or the reason for his murder. McGrath and O'Flaherty grew more and more animated as they discussed the implications of the images I had described, but I barely had the strength to stretch out my legs and lean my head back.

We pulled up to my in-laws' house, and I shook hands with the two policemen as they thanked me for my help. I watched the taxi pull away, then walked up the long flight of steps, feeling like an old man. I told Rochelle everything that had transpired since morning, and she grew concerned for me, for it was obvious to her that the day's adventures had taken a lot out of me. I admitted to her that the police wanted me to continue working on the case, but Rochelle was against my going on—she hated to see me so drained—though she left the final decision up to me.

Once again, the psychometry had adversely affected my body. I felt so depleted, so weak and nauseous, that I didn't think I could continue. I could have healed fifty people a day for three days straight and not have been as spent. I believed also that if I continued working on the murder case, I might be placing myself, and perhaps my family, in danger. As hard as I tried, I could not visualize my going any further with the investigation. For me, the case was closed.

Long after I had withdrawn from the case, I contacted McGrath to find out how it had been resolved, and he told me that the investigation had been dropped shortly after I had pulled out. Because the corpse had never been found, technically there had been no homicide. I felt terrible but realized there was nothing I could do. It was just too debilitating.

I did gain a great deal of valuable knowledge about myself and my psychic potential by working with the police, and I was encouraged once again to trust my intuitions. But even though playing psychic detective had been a great adventure for a while, its rewards just could not compare with those of helping someone who is ill.

13

The Foundation *for* Psychic-Energetic Research

FROM THE TIME OF MY FIRST RESEARCH EXPERIENCE in California, Rochelle and I constantly discussed the state of current thinking on psychic phenomena and the conflicting political forces within the world of parapsychology research. Even before my more-gratifying second research trip, we spent a great deal of time trying to think of a way to set up an experimental situation closer to home. We had been fascinated by the scientific procedures utilized during my first trip to San Francisco and knew we had to get more directly involved in research ourselves. The idea of setting up our own parapsychology research foundation began to occupy us more and more.

Our main goals were to find out the source of the energy with which I heal and to explore how its benefits could be applied to mankind. We had a dream that if, for example, it were determined that I heal by affecting force fields around cells, it might be possible to build a machine that could similarly alter these force fields and thus heal. If what I am all about could be determined, then it might be possible to synthesize my healing energy so millions could be helped, instead of thousands.

Rochelle and I had become involved with a number of parapsychology researchers and sympathizers, and we thought it would be useful to bring all their heads together at regular meetings. We began to envision our foundation as a sort of new East Coast think tank. We also saw it as a vehicle for finding other people with abilities like mine. People contacted us constantly, saying, "I think I have psychic or healing ability. What should I do?" We thought our foundation could help such people explore their psychic potential. I wanted to help them understand and uncover their gifts, as few people had assisted me.

Another goal was to help healing research stand on its own, independent of politics and selfish maneuvering. Our organization might help parapsychology research in general evolve from its embryonic state. And if we could publish the results of our testing in reputable journals, we might achieve acceptance and respectability for the nonreligious laying on of hands as a supplemental nonpharmacological therapy to be used in conjunction with traditional Western medicine.

After many meetings with our lawyer, Paul Silverman, we decided to name our organization the Foundation for Psychic-Energetic Research. We established a board of directors that included distinguished doctors and other reputable people interested in parapsychology, and Paul began putting together the papers necessary to apply to the Internal Revenue Service for tax-exempt status, which would make it easier for us to raise money for our projects.

Despite my successes in the labs and the written testimonies from many clients whom I had helped, the IRS turned down our request for tax-exemption. When Paul and I protested the decision, they responded by setting a date for a meeting.

On the appointed day, October 15, 1976, Paul and I caught the Eastern shuttle to Washington, D.C. In spite of myself, the idea of meeting with the IRS for any purpose filled me with anxiety, and I was in a bad mood. When Paul said to me, "Dean, I think it would be best if you allow me to deal with the IRS people—I speak their language," I exploded.

"You speak their language! Then why are we on the way to Washington to fight their ruling?" I demanded. "If you can't get your points across this time, you had better believe I'll say what I have to! Maybe if they'd understood our purpose the first time, they would have granted the tax-exempt status!"

Immediately I felt ashamed of myself. Like me, Paul had a lot at stake in this meeting. This was his first attempt at establishing a public research foundation. Recalling the care that had gone into the well-organized papers Paul had submitted to the IRS, I apologized for my outburst.

When we got to Washington we caught a cab to the Internal Revenue Service headquarters at 1111 Constitution Avenue, a massive and imposing stone office building. Inside, in front of Room 303, we stopped to compose ourselves. Then I turned the knob on the door.

Two men sat inside at a long walnut conference table.

"Mr. Daniels?" I inquired.

The taller and older man stood and extended his hand. Steven Daniels was lean, in his mid-fifties, and conservatively dressed. He had direct, appraising eyes. His assistant, Robert Wexler, a stocky man in his early forties, also rose to shake hands. Then we all sat down.

Paul opened his briefcase, removed two four-inch-thick packages, and handed one to each of them, explaining that they contained selected documentation of my years of work in psychic healing and research. Included were medical and scientific reports, personal testimonials from clients and doctors, and articles from national magazines ranging from *Scientific American* to *Cosmopolitan.*

Mr. Daniels opened his folder and began to read, moving papers from one side to the other and back again, as if to check one report against another. I glanced at Paul to see who would make the first move. Minutes passed in silence, and I grew edgy.

Finally, Mr. Daniels raised his eyes, looked at me, and said, "Tell us a bit more about your work."

Immediately Paul jumped in: "Approximately four years ago, Mr. Daniels, Mr. Kraft discovered something 'different' about himself. He felt an unusually curious energy emanating from his body, an energy over which he seems to have definite control. He himself is not sure what this energy is. There are many forms of energy all around us, invisible but present. For example, we can't see radio or television waves, but we know they exist. Mr. Kraft feels that through deep mental concentration, he is able to absorb energy from his environment, and that then, by the 'laying on of hands,' he can channel that energy to an ill person, usually someone who has exhausted all available medical avenues. For about three years, Mr. Kraft has worked with many patients referred to him by medical doctors. These doctors have reported that malignant tumors have shrunk, paralysis has disappeared, arthritics have experienced less pain and much improved movement."

Paul paused to let his words sink in, then turned to the documents in front of him.

"I'd like to bring your attention to the yellow folder you have, in which you will find numerous letters and testimonials from physicians who, without being able to offer any explanations for the unexpected improvements in their patients, nevertheless are prepared to attest to their veracity. You will see that against high odds and poor prognoses, many of these people have been helped by Mr. Kraft's intervention of healing energy."

I listened as Paul presented our arguments in his carefully modulated voice. He spoke of the tradition of spiritual and faith healing going back to the time of Christ, adding quickly that I did not claim any religious element in my psychic healing. Paul and I had discussed all this information in detail many times. He had learned well.

When Mr. Daniels asked about the experiments I had done at the Lawrence Livermore Lab, Paul told them that I had been able to break apart a percentage of very aggressive cancer cells in test tubes, and that the alteration of the cells had been documented by microscopic analysis before and after the sessions.

He explained that too little research had been done for anyone to reach any final conclusions, but that most researchers felt that further tests could be very helpful. Furthermore, I was eager to submit myself to the widest possible range of testing to prove that my healing energy really exists and works, and to find out, if possible, what it is.

Paul then settled back in his chair and signaled me with a wink.

I jumped from my seat, reminding myself to speak slowly, for I feared I would babble in my anxiety.

> Gentlemen, one of our foundation's main purposes is to investigate and explore the phenomenon of "mind-energy" and to report on it in a scientific and unbiased manner. We are trying to advance "psychic-energetic," or "mind-energy," therapy into a science. We hope to establish a research foundation equipped with sophisticated, sensitive equipment similar to that on which I have been tested in other institutions.
>
> I am convinced that there are many people who possess the same "energy" I do, perhaps in varying degrees. The Foundation for Psychic-Energetic Research wants to seek out these individuals and test them. If any significant effects are obtained through our tests, we will then try to train these people to utilize their energy to help mankind.

Mr. Daniels asked me to provide details on a few of the experiments in which I had been involved, and I described the results of the tests involving the Faraday cage at Dakin Labs, the startling outcome of my attempt to lower the rat's blood pressure, the various EEG tests I had undergone, and the phenomenal effects I had on cancer cells in test tubes. I tried to emphasize once again that the aim of our foundation was to explore a very promising area for scientific research, one that might offer an enormous benefit to humanity.

After my lengthy statement, I dropped back into my seat. Paul was gently kicking me under the table and, when I turned to him, he grinned.

"I must say this case is unique," Mr. Daniels told us. "Psychic healing—is there a way you can describe for us what is involved in a 'treatment' with this 'energy'?"

"Why don't I give you a demonstration?" I said, now in my most comfortable role. I got up, took off my jacket, rolled up my sleeves, and walked over to the chair in which Mr. Daniels was sitting. Standing behind him, I closed my eyes and began to breathe deeply and slowly. Quickly passing into a relaxed state, I placed my right hand on Mr. Daniels's tense forehead, and my left on his back.

Lifting his head sharply, Mr. Daniels twisted around in his chair to look at me.

"It's unbelievable! It feels as though you're plugged into an electric socket or something!"

He gestured excitedly toward his assistant.

"Him, show him!"

I moved behind Mr. Wexler, who had been quietly observing. His body jerked slightly when I touched his back and neck. After a few minutes, I returned to my seat next to Paul, and the two IRS representatives regarded each other wide-eyed and flushed, then spoke quietly between themselves.

Finally, Mr. Wexler leaned back in his seat and Mr. Daniels began to address us, speaking now with a tone of respectful interest.

"To grant this type of research organization tax-exempt status would be to establish a precedent. Public foundations in this area, excluding the religious category, of course, are almost nonexistent. Parapsychology is an area in which, up to this time, it has been extremely difficult to evaluate achievements in terms of scientific measurement.

"However, with what we see here today—"

"And feel—" interjected Mr. Wexler.

"With what we see and feel, I believe that the original problem with granting the Foundation for Psychic-Energetic Research total tax-exemption must have been one of communication between your representatives and ourselves. I'm very glad to have had a chance to meet you, Mr. Kraft. I'm sure we can see our way clear to grant you tax-exempt status."

I could barely contain my delight as Paul and I gathered up our papers, thanked Mr. Daniels and Mr. Wexler, and left. As soon as we got outside, I erupted.

"We did it!" I yelled, giving Paul a huge bear hug and almost lifting him off the sidewalk.

I was excited that we had opened the minds of the IRS representatives. At the time that the IRS gave our foundation the desired status (1976), I was the first living psychic healer to establish such a nonprofit foundation. A similar organization had been founded in Edgar Cayce's name, but not until after his death. I knew that the IRS's landmark ruling couldn't promise acceptance of my work, but I felt a sense of accomplishment, because an important branch of the U.S. government had, in its own way, acknowledged that psychic healing and the paranormal were legitimate areas for research.

Now the real work lay ahead, represented by a number of experimental designs that would materialize into serious and productive research within a couple of years. I wanted to continue my search for other people with abilities like mine. And the ultimate goal remains: to find out what my energy is, to quantify it, and then to try to synthesize it.

With this triumph of getting our foundation approved, Rochelle and I now looked forward to undertaking further cancer research. I knew the effects I had generated at Lawrence Livermore Lab were only the tip of the iceberg.

14

Back *in the* Lab

IN JULY 1977, FULLY INVOLVED WITH MY HEALING practice, I was presented with the opportunity to replicate the HeLa cancer cell experiment originally performed at Lawrence Livermore Lab, and I grabbed at it with both hands. It was still a sore spot that my planned return to Livermore to repeat the HeLa experiment back in '75 had been scuttled. John M. Kmetz, Ph.D, Director of Research at the Science Unlimited Research Foundation (SURF) in San Antonio, Texas, not only was willing to conduct the experiment and improve on the design, but also had promised to stand by the results publicly.

SURF was a highly technical, privately funded laboratory that had been delving into the paranormal since 1972. It was at the suggestion of one of SURF's trustees who was familiar with my work that Dr. Kmetz had contacted me.

Dr. Kmetz, a physiologist and a former professor at Pennsylvania State University, had worked extensively with parapsychology and was a rigorous and skeptical researcher. Shortly before my trip to San Antonio, he had published a paper in *The Humanist,* challenging the work of Cleve Backster, who had claimed to demonstrate that plants are affected by human thoughts. Two years of strictly controlled experiments had not supported Backster's findings.

Chills still swept through me whenever my mind wandered back to two years before, to Livermore Lab in California, when I'd had my first confrontation with the most aggressive and deadliest cancer cell line ever to be grown in culture. I knew even then that medical science had nothing in its storehouse to defeat the cancerous HeLa and uncover its mystery. If they had the answers, they wouldn't be bothering with me. In fact, no other healer in the world had been able to duplicate my feat. Even the late Olga Worrall and the Reverend John Scudder, among many other healers, failed to affect HeLa.

Would I be able to do it again? If I could do what I had at Livermore—dislodge and destroy twice as many free-floating cells from the experimental culture as floated in the control culture—the experiment would be a success.

Dr. Kmetz had been working on the experiment's design for a couple of months before my arrival, and he had greatly improved on Livermore's blueprint. Fortunately the Livermore papers, which I never did burn, were a great help. In order to replicate the Livermore test properly, the new procedure had to utilize the same materials—the same type of culture, flasks, and liquid medium—as the original.

The changes Kmetz made were aimed at establishing better, tighter controls. Before I even got to the lab, he had conducted test runs with a number of other subjects, some who claimed healing ability, and others who were volunteers from the University of Texas. None of them had been able to change the state of the HeLa cells to any significant degree.

When the HeLa cell culture grows in a flask, the cells stick like glue to the plastic in a single layer, eventually covering the bottom of the container. Kmetz had found, as Livermore had, that HeLa cells adhere so firmly that when flasks are thrown against a wall, shaken vigorously, even put on a vibrating machine, only a miniscule amount of mature, already-dying cells float to the top of the medium.

The first day Rochelle and I visited SURF, Kmetz and his assistant, Jim, led me into a dimly lit nine-by-twelve-foot special room with a door like a bank vault. The room functioned in a similar manner to the Faraday cage at Dakin Labs, eliminating most outside energy fields from the enclosed area. It had been specially designed to keep various electrical and magnetic waves from interfering with whatever experiments are taking place inside.

Kmetz was low-keyed: His earlier trials had ended with no results, and he really was not expecting much to happen. We discussed the upcoming work in greater detail and reviewed the experimental design several times. It was obvious that he'd prepared well for this. The time flew by, and we broke for lunch. Kmetz needed to continue with other work, so Rochelle and I returned alone to our hotel a couple of blocks away and soaked in the pool under the fierce San Antonio sun. Rochelle wanted me to eat something, but I was too jazzed—I could hardly wait to get back to the lab and down to the real work.

On our walk back to the lab, the word "contagion" kept popping into my mind. My anxiety about working with these aggressive cancer cells had not changed a bit. I still was paranoid as hell about working with this cell line, but I didn't want to burden Kmetz with my fears. After all, this was his first time doing research with HeLa—I didn't believe he would have any more information about contagion than the Livermore scientists had.

(If I knew then what I was to learn twenty years later, I never would have even stepped into the laboratory again—it turned out that HeLa was by far the most virulent and *contagious* cell line ever to be grown outside the human body. If only one singular HeLa cell was accidentally dropped into another culture or was swept across the lab by an air current, this hostile cell would take over and reproduce, turning all other normal cultures into malignant HeLa cells. So, if I would have breathed in any cells, I could have developed cancer. And even though the cell was originally from a woman with cervical cancer, a study showed that various men in prison who were injected with HeLa cells subsequently developed tumors at the site of the injection. Was it a "female" cancer they contracted? A new transformed type of cancer? The results were inconclusive; however, it remained a certainty that these male subjects did develop abnormal growths wherever HeLa had been introduced.)

As we sat in the same shielded room as we had that morning, Dr. Kmetz again explained that he wanted me to do what I'd done at Livermore—cause an increase in the number of free-floating, or dead, cancer cells. The number of floating cells would be measured by a hemacytometer before and after the experiment. Kmetz also planned to use microscopic examination to see what happened *inside* the cells I worked on.

Dr. Kmetz arranged for Jim, who did not claim any healing ability, to act as one control, "healing" a vial of the same cells by copying my actions. A second control vial would not be treated or touched at all. The three test tubes were selected randomly by Dr. Kmetz, and Jim and I went to work.

As I held the flask, I concentrated on the picture I'd formed in my mind of the cells, visualizing a disturbance in the cell fields and the cells blowing up. I was aware of Jim conscientiously mimicking my motions: When I held both hands over my flask, he did the same to his; when I lifted it, he picked up his vial as well; when I began breathing deeply, I heard him start to take deep breaths.

After twenty minutes I knew I had influenced the cells. I sensed a definite interaction, almost a magnetic pull, between my hands and the cells. Before Kmetz tested the contents of the flask, I told him my feelings. Sure enough, Kmetz examined the culture and found that I had significantly increased the number of cells floating on top of the medium. After the flask was swirled gently to evenly distribute the free-floating cells, the hemacytometer indicated an increase from one to two floaters per field to six to seven per field—a field being an arbitrary segment of the area visible under the microscope. Dr. Kmetz then tested the control flask Jim had worked with, and found no changes at all. The untreated control flask also was unchanged. I was very excited because at Livermore I had been able only to double the number of floating cells in the experimental flask.

Soon it was nearly time for the lab to close, so our tests would resume in the morning. I was sure I could do even better.

The next day we conducted a similar experiment, but this time I worked on one flask of cells for three twenty-minute periods. Kmetz wanted to see if I could continue to increase the number of dead cells with successive treatments—if there was an accumulative effect. The cells were counted at the end of each twenty-minute interval, after I reported whether I felt I had altered them.

During the first two trials, I felt I had not made a connection; sure enough, the hemacytometer showed no significant change in the number of floating cells. Dr. Kmetz clearly marveled that I could tell whether I had affected the cells. He had never before tested anyone who actually knew, before the results were analyzed, how successful he or she was.

Before going on to my third trial, Dr. Kmetz conducted another test to check again whether vigorous shaking could cause any more cells to break loose from the cell layer on the bottom of the flask. It had no effect.

Then I began my final session with the same flask of cancer cells. I knew I would have to put everything I had into this last twenty minutes, and it was by far the most difficult session I encountered. While I worked, I could feel a virtual tug-of-war going on between my hands and the cells' powerful adhesive ability. This feedback was necessary, and I persisted. Then I felt the field give way, like I had broken through—I was absolutely certain that something important would come of this trial.

Anxiously, I waited for Kmetz to evaluate the results, hoping he would confirm what I had already described to him as an astonishing struggle. Dr. Kmetz returned from testing the culture looking befuddled. He told us he had never witnessed such a remarkable scene under a microscope! Not only had I substantially increased the number of floating cells, but the cells looked as though someone had put a tiny hand grenade into each one—the whole culture had just blown apart! The number of dead floating cells had increased twenty times!

Dr. Kmetz showed me his worksheets and let me look through the microscope. Even to my untrained eye it looked as though there were few intact cells even to count! Without the microscope I could see that the culture medium, originally a clear solution, was now heavily clouded with dead cell fragments. Dr. Kmetz was further astounded because, he said, the dead cells were from a young culture, and normally young cells adhere especially tightly to the bottom of the culture flask.

During a third day of tests I again substantially increased the number of floating dead cells in the experimental culture. My interest lay in trying to understand how I affected the cells, but when I questioned Kmetz about this, he didn't know what to say to me—he had no insight to the answer. He took one of the control flasks and struck it against a composite-board wall, to see if I might have affected the cells through vibration. But, as in many earlier tests, the cells were unchanged. I questioned him about whether there were any other ways to produce floaters, and he said that the cells could be digested off the flask with a certain enzyme, but he knew of no way to produce the explosive effect I had on the cells.

Then it seemed that my worst nightmare might be coming true—I was beginning to feel ill. By the end of the third day of experiments, I had developed a fever, sore throat, and what I believed to be a stomach virus. I couldn't hold down any food. I fought all night to combat whatever this virus was that had attacked me. I just hoped and prayed it wasn't HeLa! That's all I needed now—cancer! It soon became apparent that whatever my illness, it was getting worse. The research was over for now.

Sadly I called Dr. Kmetz and told him I was too sick to continue, and I wouldn't be able to complete the two remaining days of tests. The next morning, Rochelle and I went home, with great effort on my part. Although concerned about my health, I left San Antonio with a marvelous last bit of information from Dr. Kmetz: There was an infinitesimal chance—approximately .000001 in a million—of my accomplishing the destruction of the cancer cells in vitro. Physically I still felt like crap, but my spirits definitely were lifted. I recovered fully a week later, with no seemingly visible aftereffects.

Dr. Kmetz prepared the promised report on the experiments, and I was proud that he stood behind the results he had witnessed firsthand in a variety of press interviews. The results of this replication of the Livermore HeLa experiment generated excitement throughout the field of parapsychology and in the popular media. In its October 3, 1977, issues, AMA-supported journals *Hospital Tribune* and *Medical Tribune* published the results of the experiment and interviewed a number of doctors that supported my work. I was told that I was the first psychic healer ever to be written up in a medical journal, especially in a favorable light. The publications showed that its editors and contributors seemed to understand fully the ramifications of the cancer study.

Soon I was contacted by Harry Lynn, news director at NBC-TV in New York, about doing a special three-part series on my healing work and cancer experiments for the evening news. I fully cooperated with them.

Everyone involved was very enthusiastic about the project: Harry, newscaster Melba Toliver, a camera crew, Rochelle, and I spent many hours filming discussions of the HeLa cancer cell experiments, the possible effects it could have on cancer research, and my healing practice; several of my clients also had agreed to be interviewed; and I demonstrated my technique on Melba Toliver. Harry Lynn wrote to Dr. Kmetz, asking for pictures representative of the cancer cells I had worked on, and Kmetz supplied him with a photo of intact cancer cells and a photo of scattered cellular debris.

I was elated that the cancer experiment was being covered by a well-regarded news team, and the information I provided for the show was very well documented. I felt it was about time psychic healing got its due. We were breaking new ground.

Then NBC's legal department stepped in. They did not want to subject the station to the controversy that would surround the most feared subject: cancer. Harry Lynn protested NBC's censorship, and ultimately and only after a strike was threatened by the NBC-TV news reporters for unfair censorship, the network finally conceded to a brief mention of the cancer experiment.

Harry was shamefaced as he explained that the lawyers and censors, through the editing process, had manipulated the film to show my work in a more spiritual context. I was made to look like a faith healer, especially when one of my clients who had been interviewed spoke mostly about her gratitude for my help and called me a saint. I cringed when I heard it. It was a positive piece, but I felt they should have gone into greater depth about the cancer experiment. Though the news spot portrayed me in a positive and respectable light, their misleading approach stood for everything I had been fighting against for years.

But the whole truth could not be suppressed for long. Medical journalist Judith Glassman covered my work in an article, "Cancer Treatments Doctors Ignore—They Work!" which was published in the August/September 1978 issue of *Cancer News Journal.* Then, in October 1978, Michael Brown wrote an excellent piece on parapsychology, "Getting Serious About the Occult," for *The Atlantic.* He covered many of my successful experiments, highlighting my cancer research, and wrote very favorably about my healing work. Brown, a diligent and well-respected investigative reporter, had previously published a book, *PK: A Report on Psychokinesis,* in which he had included my experiences, and has since authored *Laying Waste: The Poisoning of America by Toxic Chemicals,* which exposed the controversy and cover-up of the Love Canal poisoning in Niagara Falls, New York.

In *Penthouse Forum,* Judith Glassman wrote an extensive article about my healing abilities.

"He blew those cells apart," Dr. Kmetz was quoted as saying. "After he worked on them, the flask was full of cellular debris, bits and pieces of cells rather than whole cells." Acknowledging that he had worked with other healers, sensitives, and psychics, Dr. Kmetz said, "Nothing has been as dramatic as Dean."

It was in 1978, after reading about my cancer expedition in *Medical Tribune,* that Stephen Anyaibe, M.D., contacted me. He traveled from my old hometown of Washington, D.C., to meet me in New York. He described his proposal of our collaborating on a project involving his biofeedback unit, at Howard University Hospital and Medical Center, and my foundation. It wasn't cancer research, but still it intrigued me.

At Anyaibe's urging, Rochelle and I flew to D.C. to meet with Dr. Dorothy Harrison, who conducted a biofeedback training program at the university. Dr. Harrison, who was an open-minded researcher, organized a pilot study with some of her staff of interested participants—an electrical engineer, an observer assisting in technical supervision and analysis of data, a psychologist, and an additional assistant who would monitor my pulse, respiration, and temperature. Dr. Anyaibe would be the senior advisor and medical consultant. The purpose of the study would be to determine if and how I was able to improve the minor health problems of nine subjects while our brain waves, blood pressures, temperatures, and other specific biological functions were monitored.

After a number of visits, we had the goals clearly established and some of the necessary biofeedback equipment. The nine subjects were selected from Dr. Harrison's biofeedback study—three with hypertension, one with headaches, one with low-back pain, and the other four with depression and nonspecific pains and weaknesses.

The technical problems began immediately when we realized that my patients and I could not be monitored and recorded simultaneously because of the lack of an essential piece of equipment. With the help of a small donation given by a wealthy businessman whose god-daughter no longer had cancer due to my healing intervention, I had the board of directors of my foundation authorize an initial grant of three thousand dollars for Howard University toward the purchase of a multichannel continuous-strip chart recorder.

We continued the initial study, alternating the equipment back and forth between the subject and me. It was simplistic but I felt we'd still glean useful information. Between September and December of 1978, Rochelle and I traveled back and forth between New York and Washington five times.

During some of the gaps, while EEG and temperature probes were removed from me and were attached to my next subject, I amused and tested myself by showing Dr. Harrison and a few of the other researchers some displays of my control over my own body's autonomic functions.

With a temperature probe on my finger and one on my back, I told Dr. Harrison that I was going to lower my body temperature. Within moments, it dropped. Then I said I'd raise the temperature on my finger while simultaneously lowering the temperature of the probe on my back, and then did so.

While my knack for controlling individual parts of my body's functions according to my will delighted Dr. Harrison and the others, I thought little of this proficiency. My mind was on one of the male subjects I'd met and worked with whom I'd immediately sensed would be the only one in the study *not* to respond to my efforts. He didn't like me on sight—I could tell he was thoroughly resisting my attempts to help him. Of course, I gave Dr. Harrison my impressions.

At the end of the pilot study, three of the nine were somewhat better, five of them felt very positive about feeling much better after treatments, and the one gentleman I'd predicted at the start of the study that would show no change because of adverse feelings toward me was the only one to claim "no change" in his condition.

Although the next large-scale project with Howard University regretably didn't get off the ground because of lack of funding, I felt I'd learned a lot more about my control over my own body's functions and felt good that I'd assisted in helping improve the health of eight out of the nine people in the study. The results were satisfying, but my focus kept wandering back to my real target—cancer research.

I knew it was imperative for me to find other healers and people that could destroy HeLa. Surely I could not be the only one able to destroy this invincible cancer cell line. What good is all of this if I am the only one? Scores of subjects with this gift would be needed so the medical and scientific communities would have enough resources to study and find out how to kill HeLa. Then scientists possibly could duplicate the force fields around the cells in the same way as I, hopefully revolutionize medical science's arsenal, and access the weapon for winning the war on cancer.

I felt strongly that if anyone could find these individuals, it would be me. So, in 1979, under my foundation's auspices, I took my first step toward this objective. I contacted a biologist at the Papanicolau Cancer Center in Miami, Florida (named for the scientist who had invented the Pap smear test for women). I sent him the SURF and Livermore papers, and his interest was piqued, to say the least. I explained that our foundation wanted to replicate the HeLa cell experiment. However, this time, we were going to test other subjects who would try to affect the cells in the same manner as I had.

For the first time, I would be the researcher, along with Rochelle's assistance, organizing the participants and carefully observing, along with the scientist, the possible physical interactions between the subjects and the cells. The biologist spoke with Dr. Kmetz a number of times to be certain of all the aspects involved.

Our group of subjects for study consisted of ten volunteers: professed laying-on-of-hands healers we did not know but had heard of; healers we did know; a well-known television and radio talk show host who felt he had healing powers; a medical doctor; and a couple of others who felt they might have this capability.

One of them was Buddy Geier, my former boss at the music store, whose Buick Electra gave us the ride of our lives seven years before and had propelled me into the paranormal and healing. While Rochelle and

I were in Florida preparing for the experiment, I contacted Buddy. It was sad that if I didn't call him, we never spoke. He never called me. I guess there was some resentment lingering even after all these years. In fact, it was Buddy who was always interested in and well-read on the paranormal.

When I approached Buddy with my plans, he was keen on participating. He really believed that he could blow the cells apart, just like me. His eagerness excited me. After all, I reminded myself, he was in the car at the very beginning. Perhaps he did walk away with something special, too. My own anticipation of this avant-garde research was hard to contain.

Rochelle and I met him and Shirley at their condominium in Miami, where they now lived, and it was like old times. I loved that Buddy showed Rochelle some of the pieces of scrap paper and bank receipts on which the original messages from the car were written. He was so possessive he wouldn't leave either of us alone with them—he hovered over us and then quickly grabbed them back. That was Buddy.

On the day of the experiment each confident participant arrived at the medical center and was introduced to an enthusiastic Dr. Howard Wagner, an amiable cell biologist in his thirties who was conducting and overseeing our study.

Once again, Rochelle and I carefully detailed the objectives: to try to create any effect at all on the cancer cells through the power of their healing, their minds, their willpower—in any way they could. We explained that the same strain of HeLa, the same medium, etc., were being utilized as when I myself was the subject. We answered all their questions openly and honestly. Everything Rochelle and I had learned from my prior research experiences was integrated, and we created what we believed was a comfortable and supportive environment for them. I held great expectations and hopes for them all.

I'd decided to put the fear of contagion out of my mind for the time being. I did not want to contaminate them with my own fears and paranoia, which might have been unfounded.

Refreshments were laid out, and I allowed a half hour for everyone to relax, focus, or meditate. The tension in the room became so thick you could cut it with a knife. None of them ever had participated in any research of any kind before. I had firsthand experience with preexperimental jitters.

Then we had everyone empty their pockets and remove their belts, jewelry, and watches. The experiment room where the subjects worked was small but well lit by the blinding Florida sun, and the only decorations were a bare table and two chairs. Rochelle sat with each person, timing the trials and keeping notes of each's actions as well as instinctive feelings. Some felt optimistic about their interactions, but most didn't have a clue as to how they'd done. I observed, off to the side, with Dr. Wagner.

Each person was allotted up to an hour to try to create an effect, and some felt complete with their interaction after only a half hour. Rochelle escorted the subjects in and out and, when they had completed their attempts, I gave them encouragement and thanked them for their time and efforts. I very much wanted every one of them to be victorious.

Dr. Wagner had limited availability in his schedule, so we had to accomplish our goals in one long and exhausting day. By the time the last subject left, I had promised them all I'd call them with the results as soon as I could.

One by one, Dr. Wagner scrutinized the different flasks labeled with the subject's name, as well as the controls. By the time he'd completed his examinations and detailed his findings, we were very subdued—not one of the ten people tested had created an effect of any kind. There were no changes in the vials—not even one cell had floated to the top or had died. I was shattered.

Understandably, everyone I spoke with was deeply disenchanted—some had a better attitude about it than others, but I felt their pain. Buddy tried to flip it off nonchalantly, saying he knew he wouldn't be able to do it, but his disappointment was obvious.

More than ever I felt singular, alone. This experience only made me more focused to search for other gifted people. I still was sure they were out there—somewhere.

The experiment might be viewed by some as a failure, but not by me. There's valuable information to be gathered even when the desired outcome is not achieved. But I was left with the question of why I was able to kill cancer in test tubes and these others could not. I felt tremendous pressure when the results came back, since no other healer ever had killed cancer in the way I had. Now, after believing that I might have brought together others with a demonstrable ability, I was dismayed to find that I was still the only one.

Rochelle and I had to come to grips with the facts. As researchers, we would have to develop a thicker skin—we knew we must continue explorations like this in order to help medical science look to other possible avenues for finding cures for cancer and other grim diseases.

I also finally realized that I could never walk away from the research end as a "subject for study." Somehow, if only the scientists and doctors could measure my energy and define its nature, then I felt sure they would be able to duplicate the effects I had on cancer cells in test tubes as well as in people.

15

Reaching *the* Masses

BY 1979 WE'D HAD ENOUGH OF THE COLD NEW York winters and decided to escape to the warmer life down in Ft. Lauderdale, Florida. A few years before, Rochelle and I had honeymooned in Miami Beach, and we had frequently discussed the possibility of moving to the more tempting tropical climate. The sunshine called out to us, and my folks already had moved down there for their retirement years. Their presence created another draw, for, whenever possible, I liked to work preventatively with my dad. Even after seven years since my first treatment on him, he stood up straight and experienced few problems with his health. I also, years later, even stopped a dangerous hemorrhage resulting from heart-bypass surgery. With my focus on halting his bleeding, Dad did stop hemorrhaging and recovered from the surgery better than expected. He always responded well to my efforts. Working with Dad whenever I saw him was a loving ritual we had established from the very beginning, and he had continued to thrive at seventy years of age. I wanted to try to keep it that way. Florida also seemed a more relaxed environment for us to write my first book, *Portrait of a Psychic Healer,* by G. P. Putnam's Sons.

Every two weeks we flew back to New York for a few days so I could continue working with my patients. Naturally, a healing practice developed in Florida, and soon I had to get an office in nearby Hallandale. When I was informed that you must have an occupational license in order to conduct business of any kind in Florida, I found myself in a precarious situation. I went to the local government administrative office and found there was no category under "Psychic Healing" or any even similarly related alternative therapy. Fortunately, with all the documentation, research, and successes I had accumulated over the years, eventually I was to become the first laying-on-of-hands healer to be granted an occupational license under the Professional Health Care category of "Mental Healing." I had cleared the path for future psychic healers in Florida who wanted to practice publicly.

As we launched into the undertaking of recording my story, I realized that it was a difficult but enlightening and cathartic experience. It was as if I were subjecting myself to a daily intensive psychoanalysis as I would recall and ponder the *why*s and *how*s of all of the remarkable events that had lead me to this point in my far-from-normal life. The process was tedious but it helped me learn a lot about myself and why I reacted to certain situations in the way I had. I felt I had been given a unique opportunity to document and share the unparalleled story of my journey into healing and the paranormal over the previous eight years. Rochelle was invaluable as my devoted writing partner, for without her help I never would have been able to accomplish such a tall task. She loves to write, so she welcomed the opportunity to assist me in the project.

Finally, in July 1981, the book was released. It was a proud and exciting time. Even though I already had been written about in other books on the subject by authors around the world, it was very special for me to be able to share my own ideas about alternative healing and hope.

Between my steady referrals and the promotion for my book, my healing practice continued to grow meteorically. Rochelle and I decided to begin a monthly circuit of extensive traveling and healing, because there were large numbers of successfully treated patients that kept asking me if they could arrange groups of family and friends who were eager for treatment but could not get to me. There were also a couple of medical doctors who wanted to do the same, gathering patients for me to try to help who had not responded to their own more traditional approaches. Within a year our itinerary evolved to include St. Louis, Chicago, Reno, Tucson, San Antonio, and Los Angeles.

Learning to live out of our suitcases came slowly, and gratefully Rochelle took charge of all the travel arrangements, packing, screening and organizing patients, and generally clearing any obstacles from our path. I knew I never could have gotten to and helped so many people around the country without Rochelle's loving and supporting companionship. She worked diligently at trying to normalize our exceptional lifestyle.

As my healing load continued to increase, I no longer could ignore the fact that the more I healed, the more I felt pain in my spine, rib cage, and neck, and developed a severe sciatica condition in my legs. The symptoms were compounded by repetitive stress syndrome created by bending over massage tables for long periods of time, and leaning awkwardly across hospital beds.

It was Rochelle's concern and persuasion that finally led me to a physician on Long Island, who, after a variety of tests, said that I had inherited my father's form of osteoarthritis known as ankylosing spondolitis. I really should not have been surprised, but I was.

When I received this sobering news, I knew some changes had to be made. I began propping up my arms with several pillows underneath whenever possible (I had worked with them extended and unsupported for so many years). This released some of the strain to my ribs. However, the arthritis condition was a different matter, and there was no doubt that it was time to finally begin utilizing my self-help techniques on myself. Now that I actually knew what I was dealing with, I wanted—and had—to do everything I could to stave off the debilitating arthritis that had, until my intervention, crippled my dad. I reasoned that if I could help him with this problem, why couldn't I help myself? I remembered that I had been able to shrink the wart on my finger years before, and that was reassuring. But would I be able to affect this problem? I recalled the positive feedback I had received from so many different people regarding the self-help procedures they learned and utilized during my public seminars and in my book—and it was evident that they were able to help themselves with different ailments, including various forms of arthritis. I set myself to the task.

At least four times a week I lay on my massage table, cleared my mind from the stresses of my work, and focused on myself. I visualized the wide band of white healing light circling my body. Then, when it passed over my neck, spine, and rib cage, I saw energy waves penetrating warmly into and around these areas. Tenaciously I focused on seeing the calcium deposits and arthritic spindicles dissolving, which in turn eased my stiffness and pain.

As each week went by, I began feeling better and better. I was determined to lick this thing.

16

Battling Cancer II

IT WAS LATE SPRING OF 1985. ALL OF MY ACCOMPLISHMENTS, saving and improving so many lives, and even killing cancer in test tubes meant nothing when my family got the heartbreaking news that my father was diagnosed with multiple myeloma, a cancer of the bone marrow. When Dad had been in the Army, he knew he'd been over–X-rayed because of his long-undiagnosed back problems, and worried that this exposure caused his present condition. The X-ray emanations back then were not as understood and controlled as they are today, and his current doctor agreed that this was the probable cause.

My initial panic passed when I remembered I'd had many successful encounters with this disease in the past. I settled down into my usual confident approach and began working intensively with Dad and his new health problem. I started to see him more often and focused my treatments on creating healthy blood and bone marrow and projecting my energy mostly around his back area, spine, and rib cage.

Throughout my career as a healer, other healers and health practitioners had told me that they could not work on either themselves or close family members—they were too emotionally involved. Since my first serious and successful healing endeavor was with my dad, I'd never had that psychological barrier.

Within a few longer-than-usual sessions, Dad's blood, bone marrow, and protein studies started showing unexpected improvement and I continued to try to pump up his own immune system and visualize him well and unburdened with health problems. It wasn't long before his doctors pronounced that Dad was in remission. However, after more than a year of Dad's being in full remission, one of his puzzled doctors suddenly suggested that Dad receive a series of preventative radiation treatments. My parents were open-minded to this as long as I agreed. I still believed in the benefits of traditional Western medicine, so I acquiesced and prayed I was helping them make the right decision.

Dad was now in and out of the hospital for X rays and tests, and I was frequently by his side. But as much as I tried to oversee all aspects of his treatment, Dad ended up being overradiated which caused a bad case of radiation pneumonitis. I'd been aware that radiation treatments often can cause this side effect, but never thought it would happen to my dad.

Though I was reluctant to leave Dad to carry on with my obligations and travel as planned, he convinced me to go, for he knew there were many other people depending on me as well. He was also cognizant that I literally could not afford to keep canceling appointments, as I had been doing for months. When I resisted leaving, he tried to hide his suffering and assured me he'd be fine—he'd see me in three days, when I was to return.

Rochelle was torn herself, for she was unusually close to my parents—they thought of her as a third daughter, and Rochelle loved them both dearly. We were united in our distress over whether to leave him, even briefly. The guilt we allowed ourselves to feel from disappointing patients around the country finally convinced us that we had to try to carry on. We were haunted by our conflicting responsibilities to other people and to our own loved one. My instincts said, "Stay," but even Mom, the eternal optimist, insisted we go.

Reluctantly, Rochelle and I went to Los Angeles as planned. We'd just landed, when I went to a pay phone and called the hospital. My mother told me that Dad was having such problems breathing that the doctors were considering putting him on a respirator. We turned around and flew right back to Florida, never leaving the airport.

We went directly to the Miami Heart Institute, and when I saw Dad struggling for each breath, it tore my heart out. I felt as if *I* wanted to die. Here was my father, whom I should not have left in the first place, suffering so, and I couldn't even treat him because, from the moment we arrived, the doctors were in the process of preparing him for intubation onto a breathing machine. We were told to go home and come back the next day. I agreed to leave only because I felt it would be best for me to treat Dad in the morning, after he'd gotten stabilized. I also needed to get some rest, for I had undergone an exhausting twenty-four hours of traveling. But I wouldn't give up hope for him—I knew the next day I would create another miracle. . . .

I never got the opportunity to see my dad alive again. He died that very night, April 11, 1987, at two o'clock in the morning. I never would be able to try to bring him back, like I had so many other times. The frustration and anguish that consumed me is really hard to express—especially when you have a gift like mine. Just the week before, we had cried in each other's arms as he told me how much he wanted to live. I felt helpless—I could not save my own father's life.

As far as I was concerned, I had failed him—I wasn't there when he needed me most. Perhaps you can understand that dreadful sense of loss and helplessness—I am sure many of you have experienced it. The kindest of consoling words do little to help ease the pain. He died three days before my thirty-seventh birthday—needless to say, my birthday was never the same.

After Dad passed away, the first years without his rational, unconditional support and love were by far the most difficult period. Mom was now living with my younger sister, Lisa, and her family on Staten Island, and there were bad memories for us in Florida. We'd also had about enough of Florida's constant overbearing heat and humidity, so we decided to rent out our home in Florida and relocate to Los Angeles.

Time is what eventually heals, and I found that my keeping very busy was helpful in getting through my grief. We cut back dramatically on our traveling schedule, making only periodic trips to New York.

We rented a beautiful, spacious Spanish-style house in Beverly Hills. It had three bedrooms, two bathrooms, and even a small garden. We converted one of the back bedrooms into my office, and we used the front den as a waiting room. Basically, all I had to do was roll out of bed and I was at work. Rochelle turned the third bedroom into her own office, and, for the first time, we didn't feel cramped. We never minded sharing our home with the people I needed to treat, and my patients told us that it was actually the warmest of environments.

Now that we were based in Beverly Hills, it was of course only a matter of time before our office began to look like a film and television studio with all the celebrities coming and going for their treatments. Having worked in New York with many well-known people, such as Gloria Swanson, Lucille Ball, and Van Johnson, I was quite comfortable dealing with Sylvester Stallone, Linda Gray, Ann Miller, and many others. Treating celebrities didn't faze me, for they were just like anybody else—looking for help and hope.

Sorrow for my dad's passing still filled our hearts, but I used my grief to delve deeper into my healing work. I needed to feel needed, and each time I was able to help someone, a tiny drop of joy came back into my life. During this difficult period of adjustment to our loss and our move to the opposite end of the country, I became close with someone, a father figure, whom I tried desperately to save from pancreatic cancer with liver complications. He was film director Hal Ashby, noted for *Coming Home* and *Being There,* among many others. Bearded, with a cherubic face, this man had a passion for life that was equaled only by his love for his art.

I was called onto his case during the late stages of his illness—he was dying. He had just returned to his home in Malibu, California, from Johns Hopkins Hospital in Baltimore, Maryland, where the doctors had performed unsuccessful surgery. When I first met Hal at his beach house in the gated community of the "Colony," he was suffering greatly. He was aware that he was close to the end of his life, and he was seeking relief from the pain—all the drugs the doctors had prescribed hardly helped.

As Hal lay motionless on a couch in his living room overlooking Malibu beach, I tried initially to focus on strengthening his life force and lessening his debilitating pain. His relief was evident right away. After that first session, he was much more comfortable and hungry than he had been in months. Soon he was filled with renewed energy, getting up and walking, and he started to think about filmmaking again. I knew we hadn't won the war yet, but I maintained my belief that he would recover. Everything was going well, and I continued to see him several times each week.

Hal progressed on his road to improvement until I had to go back to New York. During my bimonthly trips, for some reason he would fall apart—he would stop eating, get depressed, and lose interest in living. As soon as I came back and saw him again, he would quickly respond and get stronger. This see-saw pattern lasted for a number of months, until I was unexpectedly delayed on a trip to New York—I had a stomach virus and had to stay in the hotel bed for a week.

By the time I returned to see Hal, I was shocked to see him lying immobile in bed, dying, and already in a semicomatose state. Grif, his companion for the previous five years, said he'd been like that for the past week. My first reaction was anger: Why would he give up like this? Just ten days before, he was doing so well! Memories of my dad flashed through me, and I worked with great determination to try to reverse the downsliding situation.

I was beside myself with sadness. I had grown to care for this brilliant man and wanted to see him get well. I was ready to fight for his life, but now it seemed that I would be doing it alone. His doctors had given up long before, and now it seemed that Hal had too.

Just as I began to lay my hands on Hal, there was a knock on the door, and Grif asked if Shirley MacLaine could sit in on the session also. Usually I don't like a crowded circus atmosphere when I do my healing work, for I find it disruptive. All the different energies and anxieties are distracting to the person I'm working with. I prefer more of a one-on-one situation.

But during each session prior to this one, Hal, who was ever the director, would have a roomful of his friends and family. He would say to me, "Dean, this feels so good, it has to be shared," and would send me around the room to the various visitors and have me give them a quick "zap." He would delight in this, though I never let on how draining it was for me. So, since Hal's treatments usually were held in a public forum, I allowed Shirley to come into the room and take a seat nearby. Grif joined us as well, sitting down on the floor close to Hal's bed.

I leaned over Hal, lay my right hand on his forehead and my left over his heart, still trying to ignite his own healing system. Hal suddenly semiawakened from his sleep and started to chuckle. His eyes were closed and he was mumbling something. He was having a one-sided conversation with his deceased mother and father. As I caught a few more words, I realized he was glimpsing the "other side," and he sounded happy: "Good to see you again, Dad. . . . Yes, soon . . ."

I now knew Hal's transcendence was imminent, and I was about to stop sending any more energy. But images of my own dad's last days, fighting for life, ran through my mind. I was suddenly infused with anger—I was there to help Hal live, but I felt he wasn't letting me.

"Hal, come on! Don't give up—come back! I came here to help you!" I yelled, already feeling the loss. I raised the volume of both my voice and my energy, desperately trying to stimulate his flagging will to live.

Though Shirley and I had just met, she saw that I was upset. In a sympathetic, motherly way, she took me by the arm, led me across the room, and said, "Dean, he's ready."

I calmed down a little and whispered, "I know, but I'm not! I should have been here a week ago, and I wasn't, and now he's thrown in the towel. I must try to revive him—it's my fault!" A sense of futility came over me, and Shirley's sensitivity touched me as she took my hand in hers.

"This is what is meant for him now. You must accept this," she said softly. I knew this, even though I resisted the truth, it wasn't the first time I had become emotionally attached, but Hal's impending passing was already hurting. Perhaps it was because it was so soon after losing my dad and I felt a similar guilt, for I hadn't been there at a critical time for Dad either.

I gave Shirley a quick hug of thanks and returned to Hal, whose eyes were still closed but who continued to smile and have conversations with his departed loved ones.

Grif's long thin body now lay across Hal's feet. I stood over the bed, and Shirley joined us. She asked if she could hold Hal's other hand as I laid hands on him, for she wanted to help guide him "into the light."

Within a few minutes, Hal opened his eyes. In a brief interlude of lucidity, Hal spoke normally and addressed each of us individually. He said his good-byes to Grif and Shirley, urging them not to be sad. Finally, he looked me in the eyes.

"Dean, thanks for everything. It's my time now, and I'm looking forward to it." It was ironic that he was dying and was trying to console us with the insight that he was at peace with his fate. Hal closed his eyes for the last time, and his face was serene.

I removed my hands from Hal and turned my attention to Grif, who was now crying uncontrollably. Knowing there was no more I could do for Hal, I placed my hand on Grif's head and began to send energy meant to calm her. Shirley joined us and leaned over to lay both of her hands on Grif's knees, but at that moment she must have strained a muscle or something, for she winced in pain and grabbed her own back. Almost automatically, while I kept my right hand on Grif's forehead, I placed my left one on Shirley's back and began working on both Shirley and Grif. We all were connected by a unique energy bond.

I had touched two people at the same time before, during seminars, but it had never been like this. With the combined intensities of Hal's transcendence and Grif's grief, the energy between the three of us was pulsating heavily, tangibly.

The room began to fill with a golden light—we all saw it. At first we thought it was the sun reflecting off the water and sand outside, into the room. But then we realized it wasn't—it was something none of us ever had experienced before. The tranquil aura in the room and the energy linkage seemed to affect each of us: Grif suddenly quieted; Shirley stopped holding her back, said it felt better, and took one of my hands in hers; and I felt more at peace with Hal's imminent passing. It was a scene I'll never forget.

We broke up the circle we'd created, and hugged, promising to see one another again.

The next morning, Grif called to say that Hal had died pain-free and peacefully in his sleep a few hours after I'd left.

This was "meant" to be his time to leave. Regardless of my frustration and well-intentioned attempts, deep inside my heart I knew this. Strangely, my experience with Hal helped me release my bitter feelings about and accept my father's death. It helped me soothe some of the anguish that had been bottled up inside and truly embrace the fact that there does come a time when death can be the healing.

Because of my experiences with cancer, my disappointments at losing someone I worked with and cared about never lasted too long, for I was starting to win more battles with this ravager.

Dorothea Chapman was a medical doctor in her late sixties when she first came to see me in New York in 1987. More than six feet tall, with a full head of thick white hair and a cheery disposition, she was an attractive woman. She had numerous cancerous lesions in her head and throughout her body. Her case was unusual, for her diagnosis was rare.

It appeared that her lesions didn't reveal their original source—affected ovaries and breast. What the doctors did know was that her cancer was extremely aggressive. They told her she had only a few months to live. But Dorothea still had things she wanted to do, and refused to buy into their dark predictions, especially after she read an article regarding my work in *Cancer News Journal.*

Dorothea was humble and unpretentious. She never confessed that she was a general practitioner until I questioned her about her extensive medical knowledge. After further questioning, I discovered she was a very interesting woman—for twenty-five years she had been a physician for the Public Health Service, was involved for years with the National Institutes of Health, and was the first female medical doctor in the United States Coast Guard. Early in her life, she had carved out a place for herself in a male-dominated arena. Actually, I was surprised that her unshakable positive attitude hadn't healed her already.

When we began to work together, she would talk to me during treatment, which never disturbed me, and would give me details of her uncommonly rare condition. Those descriptions helped me better visualize the problem areas, which were extensive, and helped me also with my hand positions. After a number of treatments, she was stronger and even more optimistic than when she'd first entered my office a couple of months before.

After three months, Dorothea went for her regular follow-up X rays. Delightedly, she told me how puzzled the doctor and radiologists were—her cancerous growths were beginning to shrink and disappear. She was getting well and enjoyed the process with the verve of a young person. Her pain was gone, and she was making up for lost time. Every few months, when she was scheduled to see me, she tagged on a new vacation spot as her reward. I felt wonderful that she had the energy to travel like that.

I always enjoyed my sessions and subsequent discussions with Dorothea, and she encouraged me to question her about any medical questions I might have regarding other patients, proper treatments, and prognoses. When I think of courage and living life to the fullest, I think of Dorothea Chapman and my last contact with her at the age of seventy-five, when she was in full remission and off to some exotic location for an extended holiday.

By 1989, Rochelle and I were feeling more at home in Beverly Hills. Our lives felt almost leisurely, compared to our many years of constant traveling. It was a luxury to be able to sleep in, even though we worked many days until eleven o'clock at night.

One late afternoon, Rochelle escorted in and introduced a lanky, limping, goateed man in his mid-forties. He was in a lot of pain—cancerous lesions had spread across his skeletal structure and throughout his body. The lesions were caused by prostate cancer, a condition I was working with more frequently, with enormous success. But now both of his kidneys were failing.

The prognosis was two months to live for musician and composer Frank Zappa. Cancer doesn't delineate between the rich and poor, the clever and the simple, renowned and uncelebrated. When this scourge of the modern world strikes, it kills indiscriminately. It can humble us all.

Frank was so much in pain and depressed that at first it was difficult for me to talk to him and pull information from him. It seemed by this time he'd been hurt enough by biopsies and medical procedures and had finally reached his limit. He didn't want to do anything but die. He wanted to be left alone, but he was persuaded by his wife, Gail, to see me. Because he knew my treatment was noninvasive, he finally agreed.

I focused on his kidneys, since they were creating the most critical danger at the moment. In my mind, as I laid my hands on him, I visualized the kidneys healthy and functioning properly to detoxify his system. I glided my hands back and forth from one kidney to the other, and then moved them all around his back, neck, and spinal column. Then I held my hands a few inches above his prostate area as I visualized his prostatic lesion getting smaller and smaller.

As I worked with him, I noticed that Frank was beginning to loosen up and relax. I knew he felt my energy—he actually had a thin smile on his face as he got up from my table. He said he was impressed with what he felt and wanted to see me a few times a week.

By the second week of treatments, Frank was not as sullen and depressed and now came in with a joke or something funny to say. His whole disposition was changing right before my eyes—he knew he finally had hope. He was an especially intelligent man, and he never talked just to hear himself. He had very definitive ideas on everything from music to politics, and his views were often cynically tinted, but I found him fascinating to listen to because he always had a different way of seeing things.

Within a few weeks of our working together, Frank's pain was substantially better. His doctor found that I had restimulated his failing kidneys—they were beginning to function again. His urologist was so surprised that he called me himself to express his amazement and to refer a new patient. When Frank got the results of his next set of scans, they were stunningly different. Before seeing me, the tumors had gone ballistic throughout his body, but now more than half of the metastatic bone cancer lesions had disappeared and the rest were definitively smaller. He and Gail made sure to get me copies of all the doctors' pathology reports, as well as X rays, for clinical medical tests had become my real meter for determining my success. Over the years, I became proficient at understanding them and had no problem calling a wide array of medical specialists when I needed further information.

It is only natural that when you see someone for an hour three or four times each week, you begin to bond on a certain level. Initially I had doubted this would happen with Frank—he had a lot of understandable anger about his disease and hated going to the doctors, undergoing their tests, and trying other alternative therapies. But his complex mind would entertain certain theories that gave me tremendous insight into the possible source of my energy—more than any doctor or scientist was ever able to. He theorized that the structure of my energy was more in the form of "light" than waves of electromagnetism. If that were the case, it would explain why the scientists had such a hard time measuring and defining this elusive energy and its effects. Frank's point of view gave me a whole new angle on how to research and measure my energy in future studies.

As the months rolled on, Frank's lesions totally disappeared and his Prostatic Specific Antigen (PSA), a blood study determining the level of cancer in the prostate, was lowering more into a normal range. He was entering remission. Soon he went back into his home recording studio and started working full-time on a new album. This was where Frank spent almost every waking minute, and they were his most joyful and fulfilling moments.

By Christmas Eve of 1991, it had been more than two years since Frank and I had begun working together on his struggle to get well. Rochelle and I were invited to spend this holiday night with him, his family, and a small group of friends at his home in the Hollywood Hills. It was a special evening because when Frank finally came up from his recording studio to join his guests, he put his arms around me and gave me one of his now-familiar back-breaking hugs. Looking well and actually smiling, he told everyone that if it hadn't been for me, he wouldn't be there with them all now, celebrating another Christmas. Frank was really a very caring individual, but I believe he chose to hide it, as he had to keep his public image of a rebel and nonconformist. Not many people got to see the softer, loving side of this complicated man. Frank felt well enough to resume spending most of the day recording new music in his home studio, and subsequently went on tour in Germany.

Another client I became very involved with at that time was Gregory, a distinguished fifty-seven-year-old businessman who recently had been diagnosed with colon cancer, which had to be surgically removed. Despite this attempt to halt the progress, the cancer continued to grow and spread to his liver. There were twenty-eight walnut-sized lesions in his liver, and his prognosis was poor—he had only three months to live.

My initial treatments with Greg went well. His fatigue and pains started to lessen, and his highly elevated CEA cancer count, a blood-tumor marker used frequently to monitor cancer's progression, dropped dramatically to a more normal range. After just a few months of working with me, Greg felt great physically, mentally, and emotionally. His most recent CT scan now showed that half of the liver tumors had disappeared and the rest were 50-percent smaller. Throughout this period, all of the results of Greg's blood-tumor markers continued to come back normal.

Our treatments together progressed over the next six months, until Greg came in with disturbing news: His confused doctors were trying to press him into having a tube or pump surgically inserted directly into his liver to deliver preventative chemotherapy. Although he told me his doctors knew of my work with him and had been given my book and documentation material, it didn't seem as though they were integrating this into their decision. Greg was now in emotional shambles. What should he do?

Though I didn't want to interfere with his doctors' designated course of treatment, four red lights suddenly flashed in my mind: *Danger! Danger!* Why mess with what's working? In this case, I ultimately realized I had to leave this decision to Greg and his family, but I did give him my opinion. I insisted he have new blood studies and scans taken to be sure this step was absolutely necessary. He was chagrined to admit that he felt intimidated by the doctors and was afraid to go against them, even though he knew he'd been getting well since working with me. I let him know he was in good company—many people were in the same predicament, but I restated strongly how I felt.

What upset me most was that when Greg went into the hospital for tests, the doctor insisted he have the chemical pump inserted *before* the test results came back! I was astounded! It still amazed me that common sense was not the rule but the exception. I had a bad feeling about Greg's situation and knew it would have something to do with the medical establishment's version of "preventative."

Bad went to worse and, unfortunately, the danger signals that had been coursing through me regarding this questionable action proved to be valid. The pump proved troublesome. The infused tube created an internal hemorrhage, causing Greg to go into kidney and lung failure and into a coma. Through his horrified family, I finally learned that Greg had not waited for the results of the blood and other tests—and they all had come back *normal*! The family begged me to see the hospitalized, comatose Greg, and, within hours, Rochelle cleared our schedule and made flight arrangements. We found Greg's family gathered at the hospital. The physician had said he did not expect Greg to regain consciousness again, and they were considering pulling the plug on his breathing machine.

When I entered the intensive-care area that Greg shared with four others, I heard the familiar hiss of oxygen, the rhythmic beeps of the different monitoring equipment, and smelled that distinctive antiseptic odor that seemed to linger on everyone's clothing. I gazed at the other people in their various stages—comatose, unconscious, or deemed hopeless.

I didn't relish the thought of having to enter into Greg's coma state with him in order to try and retrieve him, though I would have done this if it were absolutely necessary. This time I didn't have to worry because within literally ten seconds of my laying on of hands and pumping up Greg's life force, he began to revive and respond to me. He wasn't fully conscious and awake yet, but I know he heard my voice as I instructed him to move different parts of his body, which he did.

His family was amazed. They notified the doctor that Greg was coming to, and the doctor watched silently as Greg responded to my commands. I hadn't been in the hospital ten minutes! The nurses were crying, and the doctor just stood in the corner with his mouth open, stunned. I didn't wait for any kudos.

The next day, the family told me that from the time I awakened Greg, through the following morning, three other people in the same intensive care unit also started waking out of their comas! Even more interesting, during my session with Greg in the hospital, I happened to mention that I was starving and, after the treatment, I was going to go to the cafeteria for a burger. After Greg and the other three people had awakened from their unconscious states, the first words that came out of their mouths were, "I'm hungry! I'm in the mood for a hamburger." It took a week for Greg to recuperate, and then he went back to living his life.

By now, most of the cases I took on were cancer-related, and I was considered an alternative-healing cancer "specialist" because of my continual successes. It was rare that I accepted a case that was anything but serious and life-threatening. Throughout 1991, Rochelle and I still were able to keep a low public profile and maintain our version of a normal life. This brief respite from the public eye was not to last.

17

Back *in* *the* Public Eye

NEW AGE OR HOLISTIC TREATMENTS NOW SEEMED to occupy a lot of space in magazines, newspapers, and on television programs, yet, surprisingly, still there was a definitive black hole regarding psychic healing and its benefits. I thought that by now, 1991, there would have been a lot more psychic healers documenting their work.

It was October when I was contacted by a producer for *The Ron Reagan Show,* the current hot talk show hosted by ex-president Reagan's son that presented many different subjects with a respectful point of view. I was told they were planning a segment on alternative medicine, and I was asked to represent laying-on-of-hands energy healing. The other participants would consist mostly of medical-doctors-turned-alternative-health-practitioners, like acupuncturists, homeopaths, osteopaths, along with a couple of traditional medical practitioners.

When I asked the producer who else was going to talk about energy healing, she responded, "No one." She was candid and said that the show's researchers had never seen a healer as documented as I. I told the producer that actually I had been trying to keep a lower profile, but she asked me to reconsider. I said I needed a little time to think about it.

After I hung up, I couldn't help but think, *Where are all the laying-on-of-hands healers?* I had expected many others to follow in my footsteps of documenting and researching their healing abilities, but now I realized that this might not be the case. In a recent issue of the holistically oriented magazine *East West Journal,* I had read an article about three respected healers, all of whom I knew and had occasionally referred clients to. I was shocked that by the end of the piece, the writer concluded that the laying on of hands helps only minor illnesses, and, even then, the percentage of those successes were not very high. I felt obligated to counter that energy healing is indeed a positive complementary therapy in this now more respectable field of alternative healing. Rochelle and I assumed that appearing on this one program would not affect our efforts to stay out of the limelight. So, after a long hiatus from publicity, I phoned the producer and accepted.

On October 11, 1991, Rochelle and I went to the FOX studios. In a large room, we joined the other participants over a nice buffet of bagels, cheeses, and spring water. I knew a number of the panelists and made my way around the room, saying hello to the ones I knew and introducing myself to the others. We were a lively group, and our synergy continued as we were led to the large stage area to be seated. Rochelle sat in the audience, making sure she picked an end seat so that no one obscured her view. I had almost forgotten the rush of adrenaline that would pass through me right before doing a show, and it felt familiar and exciting.

I was pleased that young Ron Reagan, with whom I spoke for a couple of minutes before airtime, had read my book and even had seen a videotape I compiled about the befores and afters of the progressively successful treatment of a woman with Lou Gehrig's disease, or ALS.

When the show started, I looked around and saw that we all were dressed very much alike: jeans, boots, nice shirts, and some ties—California casual. Ron began with a general question, which was answered by one of the homeopaths, and we were off. I don't think Ron got in another question during the rest of the half-hour show, for all the participants on the panel were highly assertive and opinionated professionals, all eager to sell their books, share their points of view, and help explain in simple ways what they did and how. It was a good show, and a lot of educational, practical information about holistic and alternative medicine was exchanged. I was glad I had accepted.

As a result, a number of new patients contacted me, but not so many as to overwhelm our already full schedule. Rochelle and I still managed to hold on to our lower-profiled lives, until we received a call in early April 1992. It was Joanne Fish, the producer of the Fox network's *Sightings,* a program that focused on various areas of the paranormal. She told me my informational material had been sent to her by the producer of *The Ron Reagan Show,* she was in awe over the videotape of the woman with ALS whom I had healed, and she wanted me to be on a show about psychic healing that she was putting together. She'd been working on this program for a number of months and had already filmed it entirely by the time she'd heard of me. But now that she'd learned about my work and had witnessed on video the first miracle ever, a medical first, she was horrified that I was not on her program. She had to include me. She had absolutely nothing filmed that could come near this landmark piece of medical and video history. Her intentions were to change the whole format of the show, reorganize her filmed material, and begin the program by highlighting my work and portraying me as the paradigm of psychic healing. Because Joanne sounded very sympathetic toward the field, again Rochelle and I agreed to make an exception.

Joanne was a blond, thin, and attractive lady, open to the subject matter, and eager to get the filming completed—the air date was only a month away. I was excited when she said she was going to send a film crew to Virginia to interview the woman with ALS whom I'd healed, Nelda Buss. Already my mind was skipping ahead to the possible ramifications of this unbelievable medical first being documented for the world to see! I immediately called the patient, who was happy to accept the film crew in her home in Virginia. She already had given an interview to the *Roanoke Times,* but she warned me that they were having a freak snowstorm down there.

The filming took place in our home and in a health center in Santa Monica where I did some of my healing work. Rochelle and I were thoroughly satisfied with the production. After a very hectic week of organizing and filming, as well as seeing my patients, I finally had a few minutes for myself to think about Nelda.

I first met Nelda Buss in New York in early December 1985, after she had read an article about me in *American Health.* Journalist Michael Brown, who wrote the piece, also had profiled my work for *The Atlantic* and had included my work in a book of his own about psychokinesis.

Nelda was a short, soft-spoken, and intelligent woman who had been a fiscal assistant until she was diagnosed with amyotrophic lateral sclerosis, ALS or Lou Gehrig's disease, on her forty-third birthday. This tragic illness, which still has no known medical cause, cure, or treatment, creates progressive muscular paralysis throughout the entire body. When the disease advances to the respiratory system, the patient is no longer able to breathe, and eventually dies by suffocation. Within six short months of her diagnosis, Nelda was quadriplegic. She was told she had only six weeks left. In her graceful, dignified, and determined way, Nelda continued to exert her positive attitude by trying everything: traditional Western medicine, different forms of physiotherapy, other laying-on-of-hands therapy, and still more alternative therapies, but there was no encouraging progress at all. She continued her horrendous decline. She proceeded to give away her clothes and possessions in preparation for her impending death, and had selected the dress she wanted to be buried in.

Before she was scheduled to see me, I researched her disease in my continually updated medical-book collection. I discovered there are different strains of this neurological disease, and Nelda had the worst and most aggressive bulbar form, which not only kills off all the muscles in the body but progresses very quickly. Instead of being discouraged by the prognosis, I felt challenged by the possibilities of reversing a condition that had *never* been reversed before. Never had a case of bulbar ALS ever gone into spontaneous remission.

When Nelda and her family drove up from Blacksburg, Virginia, to New York for the first time to see me in my small New York brownstone office, it took a while to get her out of the car and into her wheelchair. Her husband, Glenn, a professor of agriculture for the Virginia Polytechnic Institute & State University, struggled to get Nelda's chair down the two steps to my entryway. Because I was running only about half an hour behind (usually it was four hours!), Nelda didn't have long to wait. Each person I saw got the time they needed, which completely threw off Rochelle's carefully planned appointment schedule.

Glenn wheeled Nelda into my office, lifted her from under her arms like a ragdoll, and placed her on my table. Then, because Nelda was completely immobile, Glenn straightened her legs and lowered her torso so she was lying flat. Finally Glenn left the room.

I placed a pillow under Nelda's knees to prevent any possible back strain, and we talked for a while. Nelda told me she knew she was getting worse because she was beginning to have breathing difficulty and no longer had the capacity to cough. She was very frightened as she told me that all the different doctors and medical centers she'd been to had confirmed, upon her diagnosis, that there was no hope.

"Well, that's not always the case," I replied as Nelda smiled slightly and relaxed for the first time. Then I began to focus a white stream of energy into her deteriorating respiratory system, her nerves, and her muscles, for I knew I had to try to stop the progression and get her stabilized before I could begin to work on regenerating her useless body and limbs.

After the session, Nelda wanted to know how many treatments I felt she would need before seeing some changes. Because she was my first full-blown bulbar ALS case, I really had no idea how long we'd have to work together. But I explained that I did know that the more serious the case, the more sessions usually were required. Terminal illnesses require more aggressive work than lesser ailments, which might involve only a few sessions. Since we both understood that her situation was certainly life-threatening, we agreed to a more intensive approach. We made arrangements for her to see me regularly over the next few months. As time obviously was of the essence, we needed the fastest possible results in the shortest period of time.

When I saw Nelda the following week, she was glowing and had tears in her eyes. She told me that after our first session, on the drive home, she felt her breathing was a little easier and she was able to cough for the first time in a long while—such a simple thing most of us take for granted. But to this woman, it was a positive sign. We both were tremendously hopeful and encouraged by this small but definitive change.

Regular sessions were now firmly in our schedule. During each one, I continued to visualize her dead muscle cells coming back to life and functioning normally. It was usually a high point in my long day for me to see Nelda, for now she always had a smile and usually a new development to show off to me. First, it was her discovery of sudden movement in her fingers while her husband showered her; then in her toes. Little by little, she began to respond—it was clear that her progressive disease was being stopped. Her spirits were taking a wide upswing, her joy was obvious, and she had renewed interest in her appearance and in rejoining her various social groups. She and her husband raised bees, so she brought me jars of fresh honey. The family started videotaping the progress she was making before and after my treatments with her.

Within six months of regular treatments she came in with the surprise we'd all prayed for—she could *stand* on her own two feet! She was able to use her still-weak arms to push herself out of the chair and stand up. When I saw this, I knew it was time to enlist her participation. I explained to Nelda that now that I was, hopefully, regenerating her dead muscle cells, I needed her to help increase their tone and strength with some mild exercise. On a piece of paper, I drew a simple pedal system she could use to work out her arms and legs at home in between our sessions. She took to the idea like a fish to water, and the next time I saw her she brought with her the contraption her brother-in-law had built for her—a pair of bicycle pedals mounted on a heavy wooden block, with stirrups to hold her feet or hands. Proudly she demonstrated that though it was difficult, she was able to rotate the pedals herself. It was pretty incredible to watch—this woman had come to me in a last-ditch effort to put off her planned burial, and now she was pushing pedals!

Eight months after our first session, she was out of the wheelchair and into a walker and was speeding toward a full recovery. We continued working with our intensive schedule, and after a few more months it was Christmas 1986 and Nelda was walking on her own. Her ever-present loving and supportive family were there, cheering her on from the beginning. They all had the type of humor that, should Nelda hesitate or be a little awkward, even their laughter was supportive. It was a pleasure to start Nelda on a self–health maintenance program rather than a lifesaving one.

Throughout her treatments with me, Nelda kept saying that when she was completely well, she was going to have a "walking party"—and I would be the guest of honor. I smiled but looked down. A few of my previous patients also had had fantasies of great celebrations when they got well, yet when they recovered, they never had the celebrations they had looked forward to—they had gotten caught up in their daily chores of living.

To our tremendous pleasure, on May 5, 1987, we found ourselves in Blacksburg, Virginia, at the Blacksburg Marriott, where Nelda and her family were actually fulfilling the fantasy they were almost afraid to believe in. The large conference room was filled with dozens of small tables scattered around a circular buffet that had everything from soup to nuts. Nelda greeted us, hugged and kissed us, then took me by the hand and steadily walked toward different groups of celebrants. I was introduced to and shook hands with her doctors, family, and friends, and they all thanked me and expressed their wonderment at the miracle they witnessed. After a while, it seemed everyone wanted to have a word with me to express appreciation for saving this special woman.

Then Nelda and Glenn went to the podium. It was unbelievable to see Nelda walk without aid. Glenn expressed his thanks to different family members and friends who had "supported them during the difficult times," and especially to his brother-in-law for doing all the driving back and forth to New York. Finally, in front of the two hundred people there, he said, "If it weren't for Dean, we would not be here today, celebrating," and he choked up. Everyone starting applauding, and Nelda kept yelling, "Stand up, Dean! Stand up!" Rochelle elbowed me to get me to stand up, knowing I was embarrassed from the attention. But with everyone clapping, I stood, smiled for a quick moment, and immediately sat back down. Yes, I was self-conscious, but I was also very, very proud. This was what it was all about, and any disappointments I'd had in the past disappeared in the glow of this tremendous accomplishment.

The small band began to play again, and I walked over to Nelda and asked her to dance. I couldn't stop looking down at her once-paralyzed legs and body as they moved smoothly and with complete control. Rochelle had brought along a little hand-held video camera, and I saw her taping us. When Nelda saw her, she spoke right to Rochelle and into the camera: "If it weren't for Dean, I wouldn't be here now." Though I'd heard it already from Glenn, hearing it from Nelda herself was probably one of the most memorable experiences in my life. This moment made all the crap, jealousies, failures, hassles, and problems of not only everyday life but my unusual life of healing all worth it. I thought it never could be better than this.

So I was especially surprised when Nelda presented me with one of my most treasured possessions—a needlepoint inscription of a phrase I often say that I'd heard somewhere many years ago. It was decorated with pretty pastel flowers around the borders, stitched with her very own hands after I had restored them to their full use. It was framed simply under glass, and it read:

For those who believe, no proof is necessary;
For those who don't believe, no proof is enough.

During her recovery, she had shared bits of the skepticism that had come her way from some of her doctors or people that didn't believe in energy healing, and I had repeated these lines to her. I was deeply touched with this thoughtful and miraculously created gift, and realized its significance: All her recent extensive diagnostic tests from the same top hospitals and medical centers that had confirmed over and over that she was properly diagnosed with this killer disease now showed the disease was no longer present in her body. This was the first case on the medical books of Lou Gehrig's ever going into a full remission. It was unequivocal proof that the laying on of hands can indeed reverse terminal illnesses that had no treatment, no cure, and no hope.

Now it was just a few days before the *Sightings* show was to air, May 1, 1992, and all hell broke loose at the cross streets of Florence and Normandy in south central Los Angeles. In angry response to the "not guilty" verdict that had just been rendered on the Los Angeles policemen charged with the brutal beating of black motorist Rodney King, a gang of black youths had pulled a white truck driver from his truck and were trying to beat the life out of this unsuspecting victim. Perhaps it would not have turned so explosive if it hadn't been for the invention of the home video camera, for the officers in question were unknowingly filmed during the aggressive beating.

It seemed it was now payback time, and the city was under siege. Rochelle and I watched these terrible images and realized how vulnerably close we were to the soon-to-be-infamous L.A. riots. Though we were in Beverly Hills, a supposedly safe section, we were still in close proximity bordering near the south central area, and we were only a five-minute drive and already smelling smoke from nearby fires.

Sometimes after an ill wind comes fresh air, and my professional life ended up having an unusual connection with the L.A. riots. *Sightings* was supposed to air that night at six o'clock, but martial law was enforced with a six o'clock P.M. curfew for everyone. For two full days there was round-the-clock coverage and all regular television programming had been either postponed or canceled.

At the time I didn't even care if the show was postponed, for we were still concerned about our safety. We just had to wait it out. I kept the television on all day, following the various spins on the big news. Suddenly, at six o'clock P.M., FOX TV resumed regular programming. All other stations were still continuing riot coverage. Because most people were home for curfew and were probably bored with the news coverage, there was a captive audience for the *Sightings* show about psychic healing!

As the Rodney King decision was the flashpoint for the 1992 riots, the "Sightings" show was the flashpoint in bringing me to another level on my healing mission. After keeping such a low profile for a while, and enjoying it, we had to readapt—our relatively normal lives were now shattered.

Glued to the television, Rochelle and I watched the edited program for the first time. They began by showing Dr. Marcy Goldstein, the medical doctor/acupuncturist whom I had helped previously by shrinking and disolving a large glomus tumor on his neck. The doctor said that for the past twelve years, he had observed me reverse incurable cancers, ALS, and other neurological, debilitating, and terminal diseases.

Actress/producer Cindy Williams shared her story of severe sciatica, a painful nerve that runs relentlessly down the backside and legs, which had tormented her for years but that had disappeared after only one session with me. The show's narrator went on to describe some of my experiments and prestigious affiliations, while various research documents that the producer and film crew had taped faded in and out. A few other credible patients briefly discussed their amazement at the help they received through working with me.

The segment took up almost half of the entire show, concluding with a detailed account of Nelda Buss's recovery. Nelda was shown before and after my treatments, and finally running around in the snow with her family, throwing snowballs and laughing. I could not have felt more proud—she had now been cured for more than six years.

We knew we were watching history in the making—televised or filmed miracles were unheard of. Luckily, Nelda, her family, and I had videotaped her progress from day one.

As Rochelle and I watched, a few other healers and alternative therapists appeared on the show, each given about thirty seconds to one minute of air time. We saw no other miracles.

The airing of this program turned people on to the idea that energy healing could have substantial benefit in alternative medicine. It demystified psychic healing and brought it to the world's stage, daring any skeptic to dispute its validity and importance. As a result, I received about 150 more calls each day, most of them for healings, but many from producers, film studios, agents, publishers, and infomercial and video companies, as well as from doctors and institutions that wanted to discuss research. FOX TV received more viewer calls to their switchboard and more mail regarding this show than ever before. It was unprecedented.

The hoopla that followed *Sightings* brought an influx of ALS and neurological sufferers to me. When FOX forwarded the first twenty-pound box filled with letters to me, Rochelle, knowing she would have to be the one to respond to each and every one, was overwhelmed. She was delighted that the response had been so tremendous, but she realized it would be impossible to handle it all herself. Finally, she hired two assistants.

Though this new onslaught of people and project offers were piling up, we still made the time to do some house hunting. After some time, we found a ranch-style house in the Pacific Palisades. It was certainly out of the way.

Almost at the top of a fifteen-hundred-foot mountain, the house had a stunning panoramic view of the ocean as well as the vast Pacific coastline that stretched from Palos Verdes to Malibu. This was a more typical "Hollywood" house, with a marble entryway and a huge living room that extended into an L-shaped dining area that overlooked this scenic view. It had four bedrooms, a kitchen large enough for cooking classes, and was more than functional to live in and work in. The Olympic-sized heated swimming pool was an added bonus that I couldn't resist.

Once we moved in, Rochelle started training the new assistants, while I focused on my healing practice as well as all the different business deals that had been offered—my own television show on alternative healing, a movie deal from Warner Brothers based on my story, and many others. Honestly, it was a bit much to handle at one time, but we waded through the offers conscientiously.

Without even realizing it, we were beginning to move into the fast lane—nonstop meetings with the top CEOs of major film studios, promotion companies, agents, and the many business socials. I scrambled to keep up with the various exciting opportunities and with my overloaded practice. Flying to New York was becoming increasingly difficult, and Rochelle and I decided that, over time, we would have to cut out our traveling altogether.

It was December 1992 when I read the first article about the formation of the New Office of Alternative Medicine, part of the National Institutes of Health (NIH). Dr. Joe Jacobs, a medical doctor of American-Indian descent, was named director, and Dr. Daniel Eskenazi, a dental surgeon, was named deputy director. This new government extension would investigate and conduct research into the efficacy of various alternative therapies and clinically controlled studies. *It's about time,* I thought.

Within a week, I was contacted by doctors, friends, and patients alerting me that they had already written letters to the NIH, supporting me and imploring them to utilize my gifts for research. I was deeply touched—sometimes I truly forgot the effects that I'd had on these people's lives.

Then I was told that *Sightings* was being aired overseas, which spurred a sudden increase of calls coming from Europe and Asia. More and more people were traveling from all over the world to see me, and Rochelle, still doing the bulk of the work even though we now had two assistants, was also struggling to keep up. The years-long waiting list I had finally managed to overcome now grew with renewed life. It was discouraging, rather than exciting, for, once again, I found there were not enough hours in the day to do all my essential healing work and have project meetings. I was biting off more than I could chew.

Unfortunately, Frank Zappa, who, before my move to the Palisades, was well enough to continue coming to me a couple of times a week, now found it hard to keep his regular appointments. The amount of time it took for him to get to me high up in the mountains, along with the motion of his car aggravating his condition and inflaming his discomfort, all contributed to his seeing me less often. I made a concerted effort to visit him at home in between his visits with me. Housecalls were now uncommon, but I continued to make exceptions for Frank. I was determined not to let him slip away from the great strides we'd accomplished together.

In February 1993, Frank and Gail Zappa, hearing about all the activity with the NIH, sent a supportive letter to President Clinton and the NIH, with a copy to Senator Tom Harkin, who had helped establish the new branch of alternative-health research. Part of their letter, which was mentioned also in a subsequent article on the subject in the *New York Times,* read:

> The reason for my letter is to exhort you to take advantage of the considerable skills of Dean Kraft in your development and examination of the merits of touch therapy. It is my belief that any conclusions you may come to with regards to this extraordinary method of healing could not possibly be valid were he not included. I base this conviction on my own personal experience with Dean and on his effort in my husband's behalf in his battle with prostate cancer.

Soon I heard that the NIH was bombarded with many other letters urging my inclusion in any studies or research into the laying on of hands, so I wasn't completely unprepared when I was contacted by Dr.

Eskenazi. He called to say he and the NIH had followed my healing career for years and would like to come out to visit with me in April at my home in California to discuss how the NIH and I could meld our research interests. It seemed I was the only laying-on-of-hands healer he planned to visit personally.

Around this same time, Ben Trainer, a husky, forty-year-old man who was paralyzed because of an auto accident, had just come with a friend from Arkansas to my home to see me for treatment. He waited perhaps an hour, overhearing all the fuss coming from our assistants about the upcoming visit from the NIH representative.

It was just prior to inauguration time for Arkansas Governor William Jefferson Clinton, who was to be sworn in for his first term as the forty-second president of the United States. Ben Trainer was a friend of Bill Clinton's. When I finally got to see Ben, I learned that just two weeks before, Ben and Clinton had had lunch in Arkansas. The president-elect handed an inaugural invitation to his friend, but Ben declined to take it. He explained that he had appointments with me. The president acknowledged that he'd heard of me and that California was a better place for Ben to be than at the inauguration. He told Ben to give him a call when he got back home so he could keep abreast of his progress.

I worked with Ben a few days. It seemed he was very impressed with my treatment, and he decided that he wanted to make sure the NIH stood up and took notice. When he returned to Arkansas, he called the newly installed president. Ben's call was returned a week later on a Saturday night, just after midnight. When Ben told the president about his initial work with me and relayed my desires to conduct cancer and AIDS research, the president told Ben to write him a letter and send it, along with a selection of my documentation and research material, to Arkansas representative Ray Thorton, who would hand-deliver it directly to the Chief of Staff, "Mac" McLarty, at the White House. McLarty would then have the president view the material, give him our signed hardcover book, and then have the rest, with a follow-up letter from the White House, delivered to the NIH.

The day after his conversation with the president, Ben called me and told me to overnight my material to him to start the ball rolling. Even I was proud when I read Ben's cover letter to the president.

> I would like to introduce Mr. Dean Kraft, a Touch Healer, from Pacific Palisades, California. Dean has had phenomenal success since the early 1970s with his practice of the "Laying On of Hands" touch therapy.
>
> I have recently seen Dean and I can say that he is the most amazing man that I have ever seen. The successes he has had with his cancer patients has been exciting, if not extra-ordinary to say the least. His twenty plus years working with Scientific Research Foundations all over the United States has had great impact in the field of cancer research and pain management.
>
> At the Science Unlimited Research Foundation in San Antonio, Tx., Dean was involved with research in determining what effect his healing and energy transference would have on cancer cells in a test tube. The conclusion was that Dean was able to destroy more virulent cancer cells than by conventional medical means.
>
> Dean feels that he can be of significant help in finding a cure for cancer. He feels that if the parameters around the cancer cells can be measured while he is treating them, then perhaps scientists can define the force field and duplicate it to create a machine to digress tumors. He also believes very strongly that the AIDS virus can be treated as effectively.
>
> Dean wanted to give you an autographed copy of his book, "Portrait of a Psychic Healer" and a video copy of his most recent television appearance. Enclosed you will also find all the documentation concerning his amazing abilities. Dean would like to have the opportunity to help in finding a cure for cancer and AIDS. Dr. Joe Jacobs is the head of the new Office for Alternative Medicine at the National Institute of Health. If there will be any continuing scientific research concerning cancer and

AIDS, Dean offers himself and his abilities unselfishly in the quest for cures of these deadly and debilitating diseases. I send this material with great hopes and expectations that something can be done.

As Always, Ben Trainer

As for Ben, unfortunately, he was unable to continue further treatments necessary to deal with his paralysis. But I will always be grateful for Ben's assertive intervention with President Clinton and the NIH on my behalf.

It was April 25, 1993, a typical bright and sunny California day, with a warm breeze flowing through the opened sliding glass doors. I had been waiting for this day for months, if not for my entire career. My heart raced with anticipation as I heard a knock at our door. Rochelle was busy readying the finishing touches on some hot hors d'oeuvres, and I opened the door to greet a smiling man with bushy salt-and-pepper hair, in his early fifties, and about the same height as me. With Rochelle now by my side, I led Dr. Eskenazi into our living room. He immediately remarked on the amazing panoramic view.

I was taken aback at how quickly he came to the point at hand: "Dean, we at the National Institutes of Health want to know what we can do to help you advance your ideas." He went on to say that not only did the NIH know about me for a long time, but the president himself had gotten personally involved, emphasizing that I must be given the proper attention. Dr. Eskenazi seemed pleased with his office's jump on the president's suggestion by having called me months earlier and arranging this very meeting.

Rochelle and I took the doctor on a tour of our home and surroundings, and it was hard to believe that a representative of the U.S. government, who also was prompted by the current president, wanted to recruit me for studies and research specifically tailored to my area of expertise. As I stood outside with Rochelle and this amiable man, looking out at the great expanse of coastline and ocean, my mind was not on the view but on the possible ramifications of the explorations I wanted to do with cancer and AIDS. Always good at boosting immune systems, I wanted to try to destroy the AIDS-causing virus in test tubes, as I had with HeLa, the cervical cancer cell line.

Eventually I invited Dr. Eskenazi into my office for a sample of my healing method (he told me previously that he was looking forward to it). After I got him comfortably situated on my massage table, I asked him to describe any health concerns. He was basically healthy but had minor back pain. I told him to relax for a few moments, and then I began the laying on of hands. My energy was high—I had convinced myself that this treatment might be one of the most important of my life.

I took a few deep breaths and mentally focused my energy into his back and throughout his body and circulatory system. Within moments, I knew the energy was flowing smoothly and that Eskenazi was experiencing it. It had become very easy for me to know when I was affecting someone or not. When I sensed they weren't feeling the "juice" enough, I just made sure they did by mentally increasing the intensity, causing the energy to surge stronger.

By the time the twenty-minute session was complete, I saw that Dr. Eskenazi had just about melted into the table. He opened his eyes and sat at the edge of the table. I noticed the telltale blush. Dr. Eskenazi confirmed that not only had his back pain eased, but the whole experience was the most unusual he had ever had with a laying-on-of-hands healer.

Dr. Eskenazi told me also that although he was a dental surgeon, he'd been involved with the NIH previously, always had an interest in alternative medicine, and was very happy to be involved in this new course of exploration. He too believed it was long overdue. Then he invited me to New York City to participate in a research study at a major East Coast university's biomagnetic lab, under the supervision of its chief, which was already established and being funded by the NIH.

It was a couple of months after this meeting that I received a faxed letter from Dr. Eskenazi in response to Ben Trainer's, regarding the president's intervention.

> Thank you for your correspondence of March 5, 1993, to President Clinton, which was forwarded to our office. I am pleased to let you know that we had been alerted of Dean Kraft's work prior to your letter. In fact, I already visited with Mr. Kraft in the Pacific Palisades on April 25, 1993. I explained the various mechanisms by which the Office of Alternative Medicine could help investigate the effectiveness of his approach and, perhaps, its mechanism.
>
> I have also proposed to develop a contract between Mr. Kraft and the Chief of the Bioelectromagnetic Laboratory of a leading university. We are waiting for an opportunity for this step to take place for initial experiments to be conducted. . . .

I had little time to indulge in aggrandizement—my days still were consumed with trying to help people with horrendous life-threatening conditions.

Thomas Hiller, a balding man with a full dark beard, had an unusual form of pelvic cancer with abnormalities of his bone structure, lymph-node involvement, and a malignant soft-tissue tumor near the spine. On November 4, 1993, after receiving a number of my treatments, he had a new scan taken. The results of the current magnetic resonance imaging (MRI) pelvic scan were documented in a letter from his doctor, dated November 15, reviewing Hiller's miraculous recovery.

> We no longer see any evidence of soft-tissue tumor adjacent to the spine, and we see no other evidence of enlarged lymph nodes or tumor elsewhere in the scan. It sometimes takes a long time for the bone marrow changes to return to normal even with the control of the tumor completely, but I am happy to say that the evidence of abnormal structures now is gone.

My success rate continued to improve as time went on, but the flip side was that my own physical health problems did not. I had been able to forestall the progressive decline of my arthritis for many years through utilizing my own self-healing methods—however inconsistently—but unfortunately my body was starting to degenerate again. Actually it did not surprise me, because with such a hectic schedule and trying to help so many others, I had neglected to take care of myself regularly.

All of a sudden, a new and far more serious health problem cropped up—I began having pounding migrainelike headaches and a series of severe nosebleeds, which created great concern. It was time for me to see a doctor.

After MRI and CT scans were taken, the doctors told me that all of my sinus cavities were filled with growing benign tumors. The surgeon I consulted with advised that surgery would be too risky because the growth was so dense—there was just too much entanglement between the tumors and the blood supply in the areas. It obviously had been taking place for many years (and he was quite surprised that I hadn't had symptoms sooner). He had no answers for me. Then I discovered through family members that this problem was genetic and seemed to affect many of my relatives in a similar manner. Most of them had had surgery before the problem became too massive. In my case, however, that was not an option.

I could not believe the strange turn of events now taking place in my life. I always had believed that I would be healing people until I was seventy years old, but now I was at a juncture where I could no longer handle it. I was greatly slowed down by my general lack of mobility overall, causing me to run many hours behind schedule. For the first time in twenty-three years, healing was physically difficult for me. I tried to hold on as long as I could, but I realized that if I didn't take some serious time off in order to concentrate on helping myself, it soon might be too late. Even though my tumors were benign, they were continuing to grow inside my skull, creating unbearable pressure and pain.

Once again I was at a crossroad in my life: Do I take care of all my patients, or do I take care of myself? Rochelle and I agonized over this conflict for months before we made our final decision. Finally, I felt I had no choice. If I wanted to stop this horrific process, work on myself was a must. Even after such an unusual career, it all boiled down to the fact that I was just a human being like everyone else and was vulnerable to human frailties.

We realized that in California I would never be able to say no to people and discontinue healing. I would not take the proper time to heal myself—if I had the time here, I would have done it already. I was certain that we would have to go somewhere where I would be anonymous. It was finally time to leave California and take the next step, which was to focus on myself and try to figure it all out. Could I continue with my healing practice? Would it be possible without continually depleting myself, or did I have to find another way of helping people? I guess I already knew the answer—I had to heal myself first.

18

The Miracles Within: *Lessons in Healing Yourself*

OF COURSE I KNEW THERE WERE MANY PATIENTS depending on me, but I also knew with certainty that I was struggling for my own life. The challenge now was for me to heal myself without any distractions or obligations of any kind. I was devastated when I learned that a few friends and patients, including Frank Zappa, had passed away while we were on sabbatical. I have been haunted by the fact that if I had stayed in California, maybe some of them might still be alive. Then again, perhaps *I* would have been the casualty.

Removing myself completely from the day-to-day concerns as a healer, I finally had the time to focus on taking care of myself. Every day I would lie down, concentrate my energy inwardly, visualize healing waves going into my sinus tumors, and would "see" them shrinking. Then I would direct the energy into my neck, spinal column, and rib cage while picturing the calcium deposits decreasing and dissolving entirely. I was devoted—a day did not go by without working on myself for two to three thirty-minute sessions.

Within a month, the nosebleeds had diminished; within three months of concentrated effort, most of the excruciating pressure and pain in my head had calmed significantly, and I had less pain and more mobility in my back and ribs. I was starting to recover and felt very hopeful.

During this period in which I was completely dedicated to healing myself, I had a great deal of time to think, especially about returning to my public practice. However, my intuition, which had gotten much sharper, told me that the laying on of hands in itself was simply a stepping-stone to another level of healing and a new direction in my career.

After twenty-three years, it was finally time for me to shift gears. I knew that my public life as a laying-on-of-hands energy healer was over, and a new life—using my unusual abilities to disseminate information on the profound possibilities that lay within us all—was beginning. With continuing introspection I recognized that instead of reaching many thousands, I could touch millions through writing about and teaching my techniques.

I had proven to myself, through my seminars and workshops and treatment on myself, that all of us are born with the ability to self-heal. I had finally advanced my techniques to a higher level and developed a way in which to share the information with others. My explicit goal was to guide others in their own journey of self-discovery, teaching them how to catalyst their own bodies' healing mechanisms and to tap into their own miracles within.

•

So, what do you do when the medical establishment has given up on you? Where do you turn? I feel that before you consider an alternative-healing option you should give yourself the opportunity to try to help yourself. Within each of us is an amazing biological system that has its own power to heal. For example, when you cut your hand, the blood clots and a scab forms, eventually to be replaced by new, regenerated skin. Through various mental techniques you can learn to harness your inborn healing system, as I have. I believe that everyone has the capability to stimulate the brain's natural endorphines, which are the body's own painkillers. We all have the ability to take away headaches or help ourselves with more serious ailments that stubbornly resist or are beyond the realm of medical control.

The most *important* prerequisite to the learning and application of my self-help techniques is *attitude.* As we grow older, with each passing year, many of us lose our childlike awareness and intuitive sensitivities. To a three-year-old, nothing seems impossible, but by the time we're halfway through adulthood, few things seem possible. Children are filled with wonder, their subconscious and creative minds open and pure, unobstructed by the myriad negative thoughts and pressures that burden adults daily. It seems that with age, many of us begin to believe in ourselves less and less and become more cynical, stressed, and spiritless in the face of life's constant problems. We find that instead of opening ourselves up to new possibilities, we close ourselves down. But I believe we *really do* have more control over our lives than we've been taught.

Remember: *Believing in yourself* is the *essential* component for self-healing. Once you *believe,* you *can* help yourself—you are more than halfway there!

One myth made popular by the New Age movement is that we create our own illnesses through some intangible misdeeds done in a previous lifetime, or, in other words, "bad karma." This theory has always bothered me, and after many years of experience in the field of alternative healing, I definitely question it. I feel illness is *not* a punishment for something you supposedly did in some prior life—I believe that *some things just happen.* Health problems are influenced by factors like genetics, environment, poor living habits and attitudes, stress, and more. Those who *choose* to believe in bad karma may experience only a sense of continual self-perpetuating guilt and hopelessness that only precipitates and aggravates the problem, and may create new ones.

You need to be *open-minded* before you begin these different techniques. Let go of any preconceived ideas that will restrict your belief in your potential capabilities. If not, you could further stifle your sensitivities and inhibit your innate self-healing ability. As Richard Bach wrote in his book *Illusions,* "Argue for your limitations, and they are yours."

As you go through the lessons here, there are a few words that I would like you to completely eradicate from your vocabulary and consciousness: "I cannot do this." These limiting thoughts are perhaps the most important ones to *forget.* They will only hamper your journey to self-discovery.

(NOTE: These techniques are in no way a substitute for traditional Western medicine. They are to be used as an adjunct or complement to your present medical care. When you have *any* health problem, see your medical doctor *first.*)

Before embarking on this journey, you need to educate yourself about your own health conditions. It would be helpful for you to have a general anatomy book at your disposal so you can familiarize yourself with the various body parts and systems, especially relating to your own specific health concerns. It will aid you also in your visualizations.

Before trying any of the techniques, I recommend that you read this entire chapter FIRST so you can familiarize yourself with them and you become confident that you understand them.

It is important to select or design a quiet environment in which to perform these techniques properly. Whether you're at home or work, you should alert family, friends, and coworkers that you are about to take a little time for yourself and that you are to be left undisturbed—and don't forget to *turn off your telephone.*

Music can be a beneficial complement to enhancing a relaxing and calm ambiance. Classical instrumentals can work very well in setting the right tone. There are expansive collections of soothing environmental music—waterfalls, rainstorms, birds chirping, and other natural sounds—and many are combined with synthesized instrumentals that can help put you in the mood for self-healing. I also recommend soft lighting.

In preparation for the "Physical De-stressing Technique," wear loose and comfortable clothing. I suggest you don't wear anything that constricts or restricts in any way, for tight waistbands on pants or skirts, belts, snug collars around your neck, and ties will only block circulation. Remove your eyeglasses, tight jewelry, and shoes. If you are wearing contact lenses that you can sleep in, that's fine, but if not, you should remove them before beginning this process. You are now ready for the Physical De-stressing Technique.

The Physical De-stressing Technique

STEP 1: A. Create a calm, peaceful, and relaxing environment.

B. Wear loose clothing, and take off your shoes.

STEP 2: A. Lie down or sit in a straight-back chair.

B. Close your eyes and *focus* on your normal breathing pattern as you breathe in through your mouth and out through your nose.

C. Mentally count *down* on *each exhale* from 5 to 1.

STEP 3: A. When you reach 1, you will *blank* the "screen" in your mind and *visualize* each part of your body *tensing* and *releasing* BEFORE you actually "physically" do it.

B. Now, let's actually begin. Starting with your feet, work your way up to your legs, buttocks, stomach, chest, neck, shoulders, face, and finish with both your arms and hands, tensing and releasing each part for a few seconds.

STEP 4: *Blank* your mind's screen. Focus on your normal breathing pattern, count *up* on *each exhale* from 1 to 5, and then open your eyes.

Now that your body is more relaxed and free of most of its physical tensions, you are ready to focus on releasing your *mental tensions,* "deflecting" the negative stress as well as the everyday thoughts from your mind.

Unfortunately, none of us can afford the self-indulgence of negative thinking. I believe negative thoughts create stress, and stress creates or aggravates disease. Skeptical or pessimistic thoughts need to be consciously deflected or "bounced out." I feel *you* can be in control over what *you* think—you do not have to be a *victim* of your intrusive negative thoughts. If saying the word "deflect" does not do the job, find other words, like "out!" or "be gone!" Whatever word or phrase you choose, it is only your magical *handle* to release and expel the interfering thoughts and images coming into your mind.

When I want to deflect emotionally charged negative thoughts, I find it's easier to use "substitution"—switching a positive and happy thought for the adverse one. Some introspections, such as the "what if's" of the *past, present,* or *future,* need to be *automatically* deflected—any outside images that will disturb your sense of *peace, well-being,* and *balance* at this time are *undesirable.* You must take the time to clear your mind of apprehensions and tensions, assisting your body and mind in becoming balanced.

Remember: "Visualizing" means "seeing" with your *mind* and *not your eyes.* "Imagination" and "fantasizing" are the important words that help play an essential role in understanding how to visualize on your *mind's screen.*

Now, for a quick practice, I would like you to close your eyes and try to visualize or mentally "see" a burning candle on your mind's blank screen. Don't look for the candle with your eyes. Use your imagination or "fantasize" this white stick of wax that has a brightly burning flame at the top. As you concentrate on this image, block out everything else.

If you can do this for even five seconds without interruption, you have been successful. Now you're ready for the Mental De-stressing Technique.

The Mental De-stressing Technique

STEP 1: Close your eyes and blank your mind's screen, deflecting *all* thoughts.

STEP 2: *Focus* on your normal breathing pattern, and then *mentally* count *down* on *each exhale* from 5 to 1.

STEP 3: When you reach 1, visualize the image of a small, circular lake with tall, lush pine trees and soft green grass surrounding it. The white cottony clouds are drifting by lazily in a warm gentle breeze as the birds on some of the branches begin to sing. The water in the lake is *so still* that you cannot see any *ripples* in it at all—it is *smooth* as glass, and there is a *clear* reflection of its surroundings.

As you focus on keeping this peaceful lake scene steady on your mind's screen, do you notice any ripples in the water? If you do, then I want you to mentally smooth out those ripples with your hands. Keep the water still and calm. Any ripples represent thoughts trying to surface, and you want *no* thoughts, no ripples. Use your deflecting technique if you need to. Give yourself whatever time you need to accomplish this.

STEP 4: Now, blank your mind's screen and focus on your normal breathing pattern, as you inhale through your mouth and exhale through your nose. Count *up* mentally on *each exhale* from 1 to 5 and then open your eyes.

Before beginning any of the following techniques, always start out with the physical and mental de-stressing techniques. Your mind and body will then be in harmony, in a place of balance and well-being.

•

The next exercise is called the "Energy Circulation Technique," and it is for everyone. It is especially useful to *healthy* people who want to maintain their wellness and work preventatively. I believe it also aids the *circulatory* and the *immune systems* in functioning optimally, and boosts your energy level to help combat fatigue. This technique takes only ten minutes a day of your time. Utilize it during the second part of your day, when your natural energy level is running low.

The Energy Circulation Technique

STEP 1: Create your peaceful and quiet environment.

STEP 2: Do the Physical De-stressing Technique.

STEP 3: Do the Mental De-stressing Technique.

STEP 4: **A.** Focus on your normal breathing pattern, and then mentally count *down* on *each exhale* from 5 to 1.

B. As soon as you reach 1, visualize the white image of your body in your mind's dark, blank screen. Once you mentally "see" this clearly, visualize a wide four-inch band of white healing light. It begins at the top of your head, flows down the left side of your head on your body's image, and moves slowly along your body. You will move this light by *propelling* and *controlling* it with your *breathing*: As you *inhale,* the light moves *slowly,* and as you *exhale,* it moves more *quickly,* until it finally en-

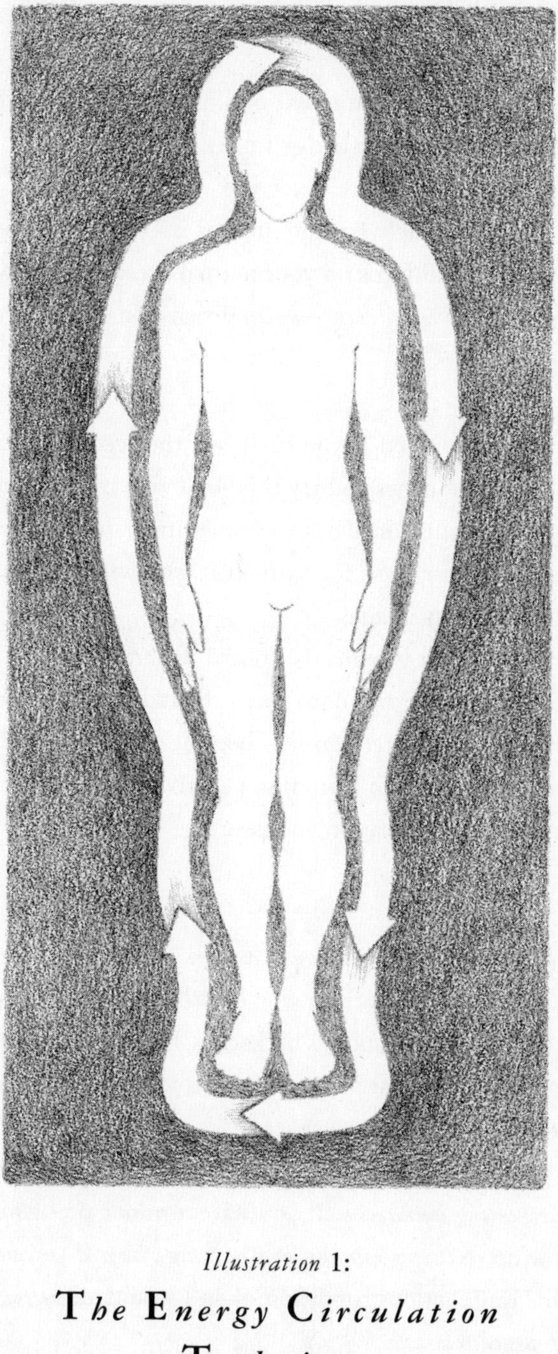

Illustration 1:
The Energy Circulation Technique

circles your entire body's outline, returns to your head, and begins to flow around *again* (see illustration 1).

Try to imagine a warm sensation flowing along with the light as it makes its way around your body's image.

STEP 5: After approximately ten minutes, or *when you feel satisfied,* blank your mind's screen and focus on your normal breathing. Now mentally count *up* from 1 to 5 on *each exhale.* When you reach 5, open your eyes.

Do not be discouraged if you can't feel the accompanying heat or warmth the first few times you try this. In a way, it's like patting your head and rubbing your stomach at the same time—it takes coordination and practice. Have patience, for without it, you will find it difficult to focus and to create *any* image!

In the beginning, it is perfectly normal if your concentration wavers and your focus fades in and out. You will find that the more you do these techniques, the better you will become at them and the easier it will be for you to get rid of intruding negative thoughts, focus on, and hold any image or visualization you desire.

•

The next exercise we will do is called the "Self-healing Visualization Technique." It is for those of you who have health problems that Western medicine cannot help, such as backaches, headaches, cramps, or more serious conditions like poor immunity, neurological or circulatory problems, severe arthritis, and even cancer.

With this upcoming technique, you will try to *stimulate your own body's innate healing mechanism.* If you have a minor problem, then you should allow up to *twenty minutes, once or twice a day.* If you need to concentrate on a more serious condition, then I would allow *thirty minutes, up to three times each day.*

The Self-healing Visualization Technique

STEP 1: Create your optimal quiet and relaxing environment.

STEP 2: Do the Physical De-stressing Technique.

STEP 3: Do the Mental De-stressing Technique, and deflect all thoughts.

STEP 4: Focus on your breathing and count *down* from 5 to 1 on *each exhale*. When you reach 1, *blank* out your mind's screen and visualize your body's image in white contrast.

STEP 5: Circulate the white band of light several times around your body's image, until you feel comfortable that you can mentally control the image and the movement of the light with your breathing.

STEP 6: Now, focus on your specific problem area. When the white band of light reaches it, *expand* it to *twice* its width over that area (see illustration 2).

For example, if you have a *backache,* then you will first visualize the light *expanding* into your back area. *Hold* that image for *five seconds* on your mind's screen. Right after that, visualize a *close-up* image of your back's tight and knotted muscles being *penetrated by waves of healing energy,* and then visualize these muscles *smoothing out,* releasing and relaxing. While you are doing this, try to *create* and *feel* a warmth or heat sensation in the same area. *Be patient.* The more you practice, the more proficient you will become.

STEP 7: After *holding* this image for another *five seconds,* allow your band of white light to continue around your body for another revolution. With

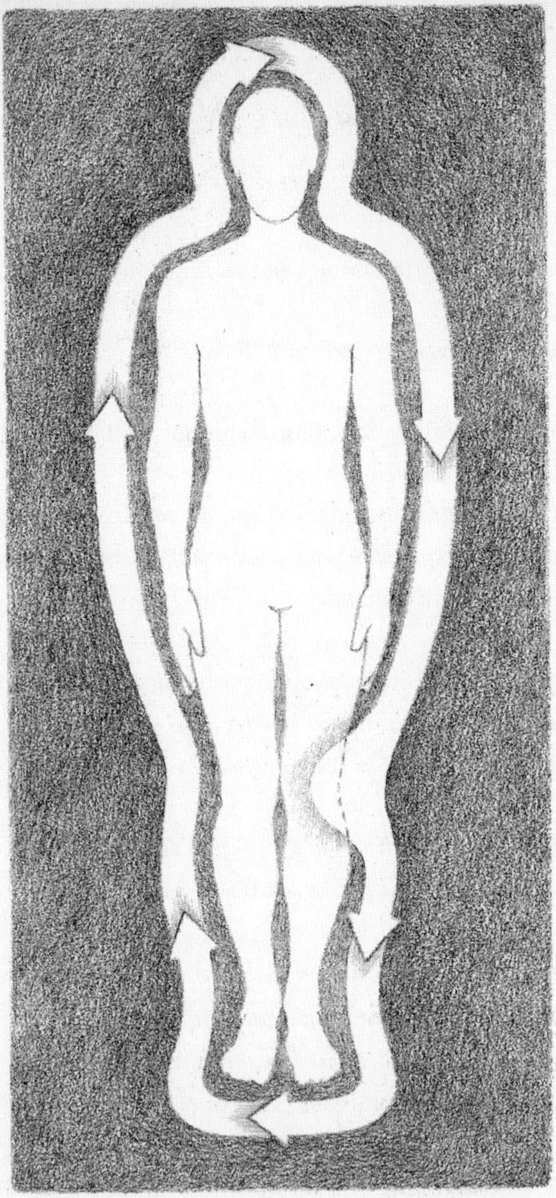

Illustration 2:

The Self-Healing Visualization Technique

Focus on the band of white healing light, and mentally EXPAND it to DOUBLE ITS WIDTH over the afflicted area.

every revolution, you should spend *five seconds* on the white light *expansion,* and then *five seconds* on the *close-up* of, for instance, your back and spinal column. This same process is used for *all* illnesses, minor or chronic. The *difference* is in your *close-up* visualization of the problem.

If you have a *bone spur* on your foot, elbow, or ankle, the *close-up* image will be of the spur *dissolving* right before your eyes.

If you suffer from *menstrual cramps,* your specific *close-up* visualization would be of energy waves, like those you see when you look at a very hot road and the heat waves emanate from the tar pavement. Visualize the waves *penetrating into your pelvis and lower abdomen.*

If you have a *headache,* then you would imagine the same healing energy waves penetrating and then releasing tension in the *area of your head* where you feel the pain.

Minor problems other than these, such as pain, fatty tumors, or cramped muscles anywhere, can be handled in a similar manner.

For more serious health problems, such as *brain, breast, ovarian, or prostate tumors,* you should visualize *penetrating healing energy waves going into the lesion.* (Here it would be helpful if you knew the exact location and measurements of the growth.) You would then "see" or imagine on your mind's screen this mass of *abnormal cells shrinking and dissolving.*

If your problem is *neurological,* imagine the *healing waves of energy penetrating through your entire spinal column.*

For *immune disorders,* your main visualization would be the *expansion* of the white light that encircles your body's image to *double* its width as it travels *around the entire body,* synchronized with your normal breathing pattern. If you have other complications, you can alternate different *close-up* visualizations by sending healing energy waves into those areas.

STEP 8: After you are satisfied with your session, blank your mind's screen and then focus on your normal breathing pattern for a few moments. Now mentally count *up* on *each exhale* from 1 to 5, and open your eyes.

If, after working with these techniques over a period of a month or so, you find your condition has not improved at all, now might be the time to consider researching an alternative healing therapy.

If you have received *any* favorable benefit from working on yourself, then *continue* to do these techniques to see if you can improve on those positive changes.

If you feel you have grasped the concepts and have been able to effect encouraging results, you will definitely be interested in what follows.

19

The Infinite Connection:

Helping Others Through Loving Touch

THE LAYING ON OF HANDS IS NOT A NEW IDEA OR therapy—it has been around for thousands of years. Throughout the millenniums, people from all corners of the world have laid on hands to help the sick—from the tribal shaman to the loving mother who tenderly touches her child's feverish head with her hand and brings the temperature down. I believe we *all* are born with this *natural and innate gift* to help stimulate *someone else's* own healing mechanism.

I began a number of public seminars and lectures across the country in 1974 to teach lay people, a number of psychologists, and medical doctors my own healing methods. They were so palatable to the physicians that they frequently invited me to share my ideas at various hospitals and medical centers.

In 1976, Michael O. Smith, M.D., director of the Drug Detoxification Unit at Lincoln Hospital in the Bronx, New York, invited me to teach my methods to a group of medical doctors in the unit, who then utilized them on their patients. Today, this hospital is still successfully employing my laying-on-of-hands techniques, as well as acupuncture and other alternative therapies, and has one of the highest cure rates of all detox units in the U.S. After conducting these seminars with doctors and lay people during the last two decades, and seeing the amazing results and beneficial changes they were able to stimulate, I realized the need for disseminating my techniques to the public.

This procedure can be helpful for a number of minor ailments that there are no cures for, however it is *really meant* to be used on *loved ones* who are ill, have *exhausted all medical avenues,* and basically *have no hope left.* I have always believed that people should give medical science the *first* chance to help them with their health problems. When people have *any* medical emergencies at all, such as broken bones, severe pains, infections, fevers, etc., they need to go to doctors immediately—*not* alternative healers!

After learning this methodology and before attempting to help someone, you should get some medical history from them, for it will be beneficial later when you lay on hands and visualize the health problem. It will aid you also when teaching your loved one how to visualize properly.

I have found that it is very important that you *exude confidence*—if you are *not* self-assured, then you *should not* be doing this in the first place. All people are sensitive, especially the ill, and if you are not optimistic and sure of yourself, the person will pick up on it and perhaps be uncomfortable. Furthermore, you should attempt a healing only when you *really believe* you might be able to help stimulate and catalyst the ill person's own healing system and, of course, when you comprehend all of the steps, hand positions, and visualizations completely.

Not everyone is meant to, or even likes to, touch others. As well, there are people who like to be touched, and those who do not. It's important that you don't push yourself on your loved ones but rather suggest to them that since the doctors couldn't help, maybe they would like to let you try the laying on of hands to stimulate their own healing systems. Be straightforward and tell them you can offer no guarantees that it will help, but it certainly cannot hurt to try.

If the ill person is not sure, *do not do it*! Go forward only if the person is enthusiastic about the idea.

Here are some other situations when you *do not* want to lay on hands.

1. If you don't thoroughly know and completely understand all of the self-help and laying-on-of-hands techniques
2. The person has severe pain *anywhere* that is undiagnosed
3. The person does not want, or like, to be touched
4. The person *does not know or understand* what you are going to try to do
5. The person's body is sensitive to touch or any pressure
6. The person is hooked up to delicate life-saving equipment, such as respirators, IV drips, etc., and you can't get near her or him to touch without mistakenly pulling out a plug or disturbing the instruments
7. If any family members present are *hostile* to you or your desire to try to help, or are *blatantly unsupportive* toward your attempted ministrations
8. *When you are sick or not feeling well.* If you have a cold or flu, do not even think about working with someone. You could easily pass on the cold or flu, and because that person has a weakened immune system, he or she could develop possibly life-threatening pneumonia. Also, if you are not fit to do the laying on of hands, then, in the process of trying to help someone, you could get very drained and feel even worse.
9. If the person you want to treat has a *contagious or infectious condition,* like a cold, flu, hepatitis, or conjunctivitis (pink eye). Postpone your healing attempt to a time when the infection is *no longer communicable.* Even if you don't get sick yourself, you could be a "carrier" to another person.

Once again, it is essential that you thoroughly understand, and even memorize, all the techniques *before* even attempting to apply them. Also, if you care enough about this person to want to try to help them, then they also deserve to learn the physical and mental de-stressing techniques and the Self-healing Visualization Technique as well, so that while you are working on them, they can do these visualizations. It will give them a good headstart on helping them stimulate *their own* healing mechanisms.

•

After establishing a quiet, peaceful, dimly lit environment, allow yourself *twenty minutes' preparation* time before attempting to help someone—you must first prepare your own "instrument." It is essential that your mind and body be in harmony and synergistically clear, calm, and free of all mental and physical tensions.

You will need to prepare yourself for your interaction using the physical and mental de-stressing techniques. After that, do the Energy Circulation Technique for ten minutes—This will act as a preventative step for keeping your *own* body's healing system strong and free of any negativity that you could pick up from the ill person. I believe a very high-level and positive energy field, and a positive attitude, will burn away any stray accumulative negativity.

The next step is to prepare the loved one for what you are about to attempt. You must explain that what you are going to do is an *experiment*—an undertaking to *try* to stimulate the body's natural healing system. Get a rundown from the person about his or her medical diagnosis, and be sure all medical routes have been exhausted.

The next step is to make the person comfortable in a firm, straight-back chair. Then *wash your hands* for at least twelve seconds, using hot water and plenty of soap. This will help kill any germs or bacteria.

Once you've thoroughly cleaned your hands and the person you are about to work with is sitting comfortably, enhance the relaxing atmosphere with instrumental, classical, or environmental music. You will find it important to have a watch with a timer in order to time your treatment—you will probably get so involved in what you're doing that you may lose all conception of time.

You need to build up your treatment time gradually, and divide the extra time between all the positions related to the specific health problem you're working with. Some people feel comfortable doing this for five minutes, others prefer twenty minutes. If after only three minutes of treating you feel exhausted, then that's your signal to stop. Do not feel discouraged—this happens to many people. You have to consider your own body's position. If you become uncomfortable or achy, you definitely need to stop.

Like any other discipline, the more you practice, the more adept you will become without draining yourself. Eventually you will be able to build up to twenty minutes. Never exceed that amount of time. Remember: It is not the *amount* of time that's important, but the feeling that you have made a *connection* and had a *quality* session.

•

Now, with your loved one comfortable and you understanding the diagnosis, have the person close his eyes. Thoroughly explain and guide the person through the physical and mental de-stressing techniques. Once he comprehends these simple relaxing exercises, talk him through his own specific Self-healing Visualization Technique, which he will do while you're working on him as well as at home himself (see chapter 18). Even if the person seems to have a problem in grasping the technique right away, explain that just by *learning and trying it* he *is* calming and relaxing himself and is a better receptor to your ministrations. It's time to encourage the person to learn how he can help *himself,* too.

I call my laying on of hands technique "Infinite Connection," for when I did my very first healings, I got an involuntary image on my mind's screen of a figure-eight lying on its side.

Then I saw what appeared to be a band of white light flowing along this path from one side to the other. One side seemed to be the *healer sending* the energy, and the other side was the *healee receiving* the energy. From then on, I have used this infinity symbol to represent the laying on of hands to others. It is similar to a car with a weak battery getting a boost or a charge from a stronger one.

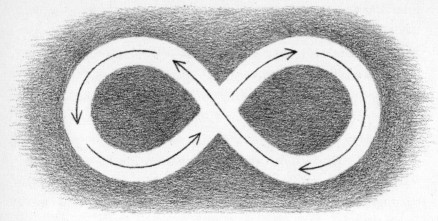

Illustration 3:
The Infinite Connection

I will now take you step by step, diagram by diagram, through the laying on of hands as you try to help a loved one who has exhausted all medical routes regarding these specific illnesses:

1. Chronic fatigue syndrome (CFS)
2. Headaches
3. Backaches
4. Menstrual cramps and premenstrual syndrome (PMS)

I will guide you in what you will do and visualize, as well as what image your loved one should visualize during the process. You will be shown where and how to place or hold your hands for the specific problem area. And when you do touch the person, don't be heavy-handed—a light, gentle touch is what's desirable.

After your session, I strongly recommend that you *do not* question the person as to how he/she feels—it is much too soon. *If* the person has felt something, it's better for him or her to tell you, without provocation.

Also, I encourage family members to do the same and not pester the person about the session. The ill person will need time to absorb this experience and process the information, letting it resonate properly within his or her body. The timing is relative—some people may be eager to share their feelings, others reluctant. Give them whatever space they need.

If the person did feel something encouraging or did benefit from your treatment, he will be the *first* to tell you and ask for more sessions. Let *the person* be the one to ask you. If he is enthusiastic and you were not drained from doing this, then I would suggest continuing the treatment once a week until the person improves.

Chronic Fatigue Syndrome

Make sure your loved one has gone through the proper medical tests to eliminate other serious illnesses that may mimic chronic fatigue syndrome.

Wash your hands.
Seat your loved one in a straight-back chair.
Play instrumental music, if desired.
Adjust lighting.

STEP 1: Teach and take the person through the Physical De-stressing Technique.

STEP 2: Teach and take the person through the Mental De-stressing Technique.

STEP 3: Teach, practice, and take the person through the following Self-healing Visualization for CFS. I believe the best "visualization" for this systemic condition is the Energy Circulation Technique (see chapter 18).

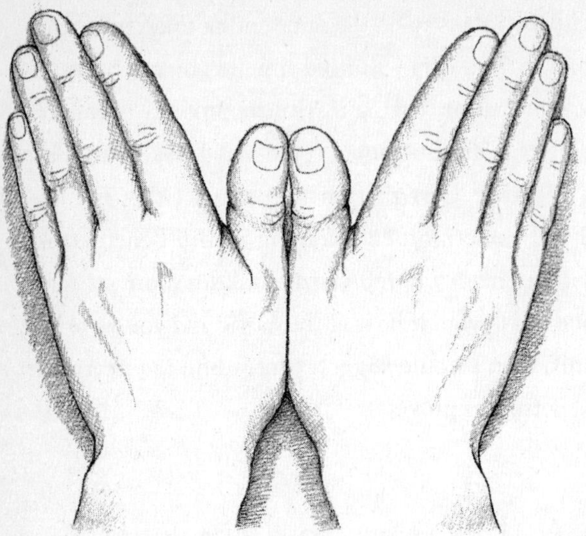

Illustration 4:
The "Butterfly" Position

Illustration 5:
"Butterfly" ON forehead and temples

Illustration 6:
"Butterfly" 1 to 3 inches AWAY from forehead

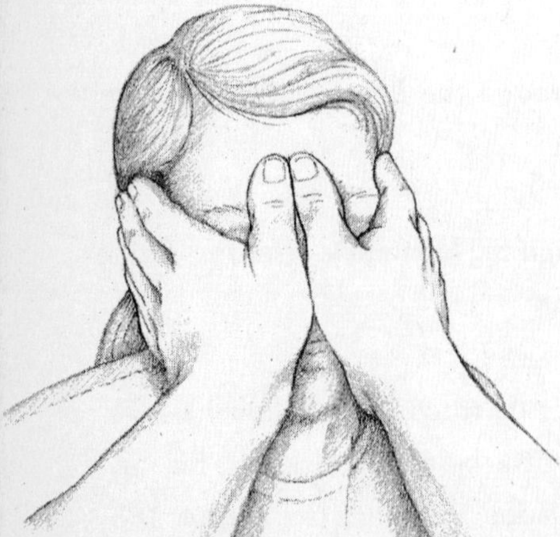

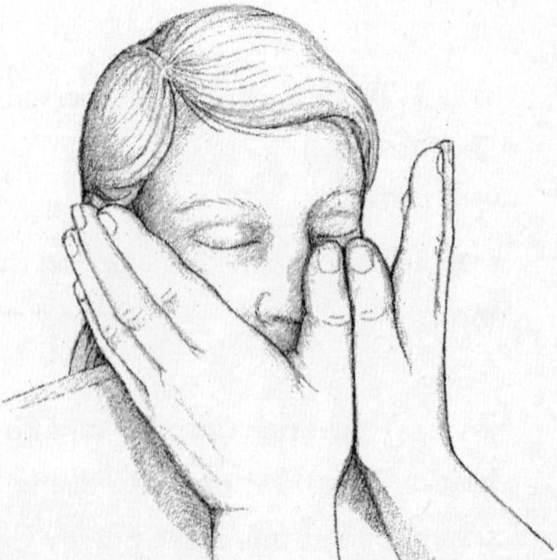

However, the person should visualize the white band of light expanding to *double* its width around the *entire body's image.*

You and your loved one will do this visualization at the same time you are doing the hand positions.

STEP 4: Have your loved one close his eyes and focus on his normal breathing pattern. Have him mentally count *down* from 5 to 1 on *each exhale,* then have him blank his mind's "screen." Tell him to begin his specific visualization for chronic fatigue syndrome.

Put your fingers together with both thumbs touching each other, in the "butterfly" position (see illustration 4). Then, place both thumbs *gently* on the "third eye" (mid-forehead area) and, with the rest of your fingers, lightly touch the temples (see illustration 5).

Once you've gently placed your hands, *hold* them here for 5 seconds.

Then *raise* both hands simultaneously to a height of 1 to 3 inches *away* from the person's head (see illustration 6). *Hold* that position for about 60 seconds.

Now, bring your hands back down lightly onto the person's head at the same original touch points (illustration 5). *Hold* your hands in that position for 5 seconds, and then lift them again.

Relax your hands and arms by your sides. Tense and release them a few times.

STEP 5: Stand at the person's side and lightly place your *left* hand, fingers touching, on the person's forehead. *At the same time,* place your *right* hand, fingers touching, on the mid-spine and shoulder blades (see illustration 7). *Hold* these positions for 5 seconds.

Then, *raise* both your hands 1 to 3 inches *away* from the forehead and back (see illustration 8). Keep both hands in this above-body position for approximately 60 seconds.

Now, bring both hands back down to the original touch-point areas again (illustration 7), and *hold* for 5 seconds.

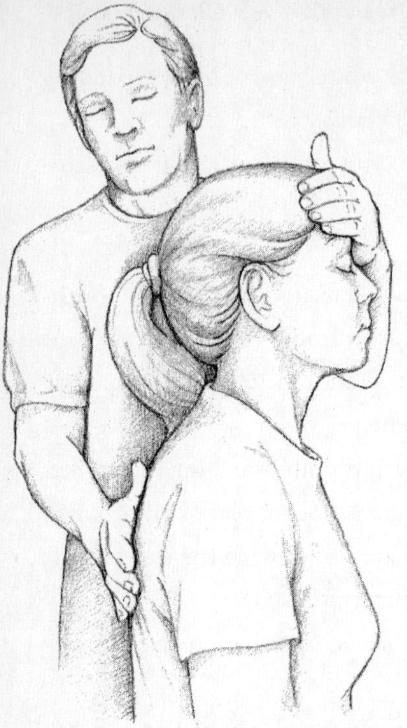

Illustration 7:

Hands ON forehead and mid-back

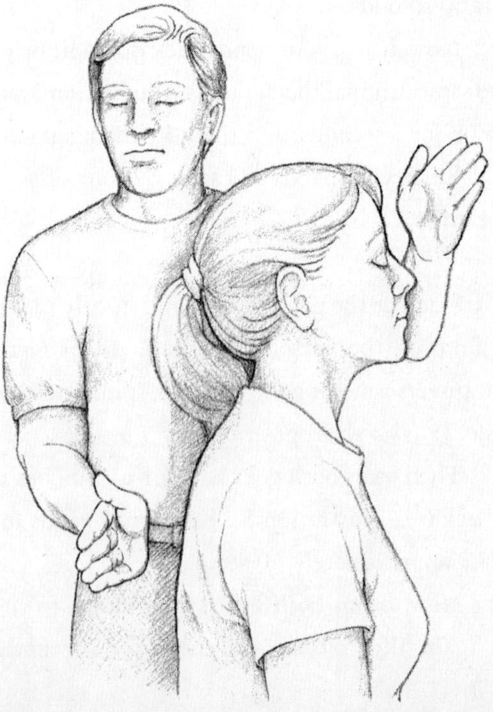

Illustration 8:

Hands 1 to 3 inches AWAY from forehead and mid-back

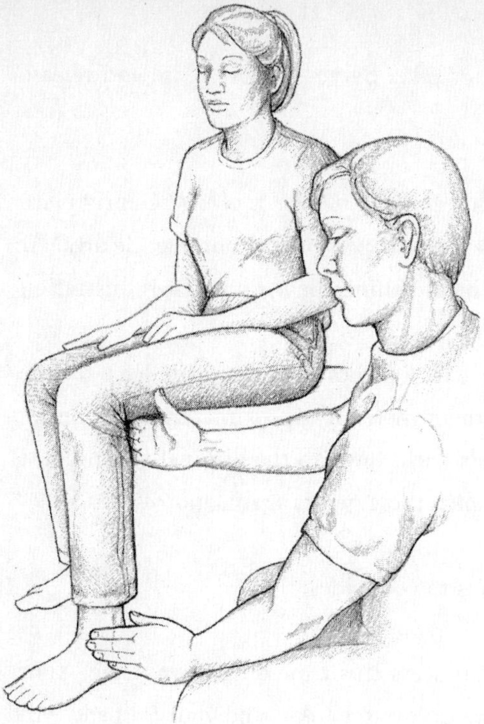

Illustration 9:
Hands ON left ankle and behind left knee

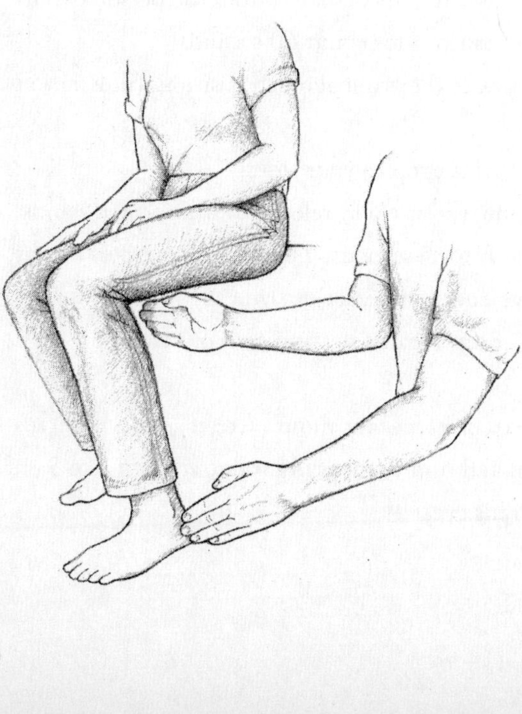

Illustration 10:
Hands 1 to 3 inches AWAY from left ankle and left knee

Let your arms and hands relax by your sides. Tense and release them a few times.

STEP 6: Here you will have to kneel down. *Do not bend over!* Gently place your *left* hand, fingers together, on the person's *left* outer ankle area. *At the same time,* place your *right* hand behind the *left* knee (see illustration 9). *Hold* for 5 seconds.

Now, *raise* your hands 1 to 3 inches *away* from the leg's surface (see illustration 10) and *hold* them there for approximately 60 seconds.

Then, bring both hands back down to the original touch-point areas (illustration 9), gently touch these points again, and *hold* for 5 seconds.

Slowly lower your hands to your sides.

STEP 7: Now, repeat the exact process this time on the right leg. Your *right* hand will be touching the *right* outer ankle, and your *left* hand will be touching the back of the *right* knee (see illustration 11). *Hold* for 5 seconds.

Next, *raise* both hands 1 to 3 inches *away* from the person (see illustration 12). *Hold* these positions for about 60 seconds.

Bring both hands back to the original touch positions (illustration 11) and *hold* for 5 seconds.

Let your hands and arms drop to your sides.

Finally, stand up slowly, tense and release your arms and hands, and *shake both hands vigorously* for 5 seconds. This shaking process acts as an "accumulative negative-energy releaser" so you won't pick up any stray negativity. Take in 3 deep breaths, letting each out slowly.

STEP 8: Now, have your loved one *blank* his mind's screen and focus on his normal breathing pattern. Tell him to mentally count *up* from 1 to 5 on *each exhale,* and then open his eyes.

Wash your hands.

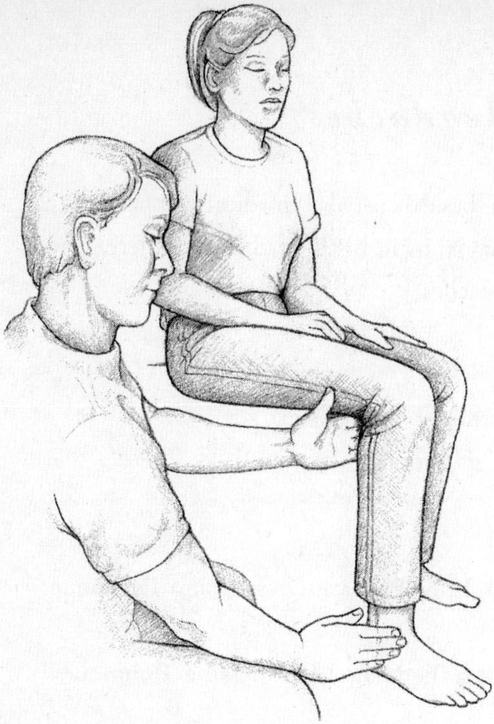

Illustration 11:

Hands ON right ankle and behind right knee

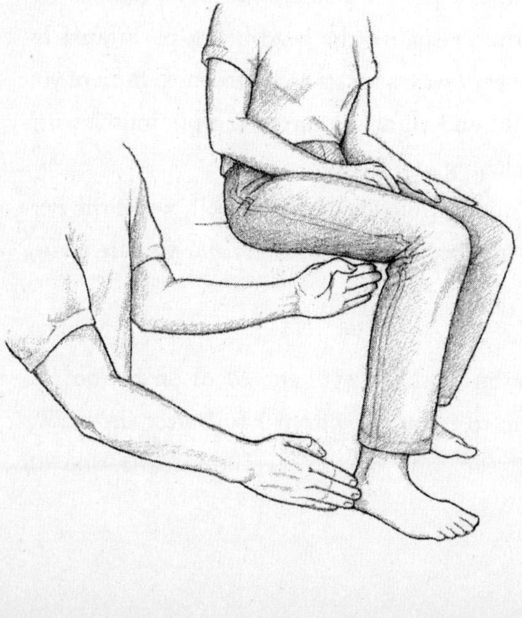

Illustration 12:

Hands 1 to 3 inches AWAY from right ankle and right knee

Headaches

First, ascertain that the person has exhausted all medical avenues and that he is not having some *unusual* pains in his head that are different from or unrelated to everyday headaches.

Wash your hands.
Seat your loved one in a straight-back chair.
Play instrumental music, if desired.
Adjust lighting.

STEP 1: Take the person through the Physical De-stressing Technique.

STEP 2: Take the person through the Mental De-stressing Technique.

STEP 3: Start the Self-help Visualization Technique. Instruct the person to mentally "see" the band of white light flowing around his own body's image on his mind's "screen" and then *expanding* to *double its width* over the painful area of the head. The person should *hold* this *expanded* white light for 5 seconds, and then visualize the head being penetrated by soothing, warm, healing energy waves for *another* 5 seconds. Both of you should visualize the painful and tightly knotted temple muscles unknotting, releasing, and relaxing.

Do the Self-help Visualization Technique as well, while the person is doing it. Focus on this specific visualization *while* you are laying on hands.

STEP 4: Now, have the person close his eyes and focus on his normal breathing pattern. Tell him to count *down* from 5 to 1 after *each exhale,* then *blank* his mind's "screen" and do the specific visualization for headaches.

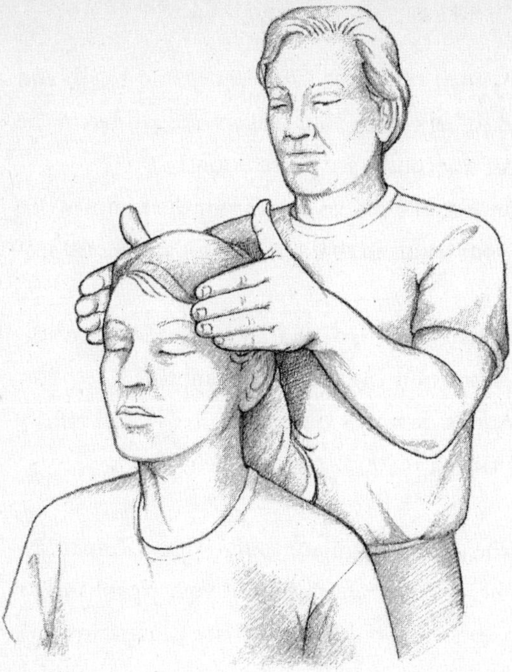

Illustration 13:
Hands ON temples

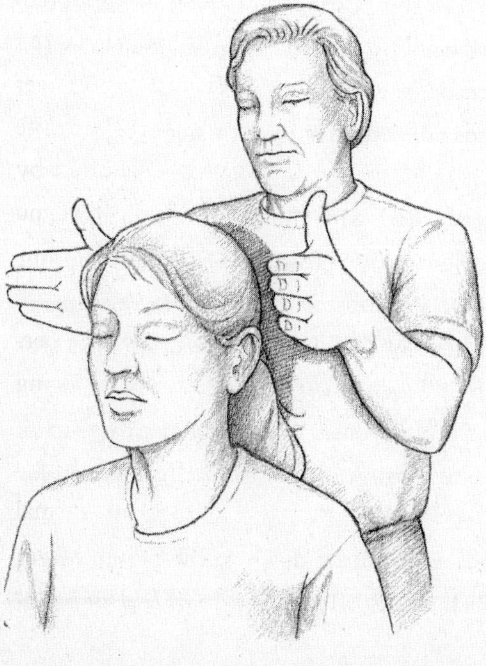

Illustration 14:
Hands 1 to 3 inches
AWAY from temples

STEP 5: Now, stand behind your loved one. With your thumbs up and your other fingers together, lightly place your fingers and palms on the person's temples and *hold* for 5 seconds (see illustration 13).

Gently *raise* both hands 1 to 3 inches *away* from the temples (see illustration 14). *Hold* both your hands in that position for at least 60 seconds.

Then, bring both hands gently back to the temples in the original touch-point position (illustration 13) and *hold* for another 5 seconds.

Slowly bring your hands down to your sides. Tense and release your arms and hands a few times.

STEP 6: Stand to the side of the person and place your *left* hand, fingers together, on the person's forehead. *At the same time,* put your *right* hand on the person's mid-spine between the shoulder blades (see illustration 15). *Hold* those positions for 5 seconds.

Now, *raise* both your hands 1 to 3 inches *away* from the person's body (see illustration 16) and *hold* this positions for about 60 seconds.

Then, gently lower both hands to the same original point areas (illustration 15) and *hold* for 5 seconds.

Let your arms and hands fall and relax by your sides.

STEP 7: Stand in front of the person and, with thumbs touching and your other fingers together in the "butterfly" position, place both thumbs gently on the person's third eye (mid-forehead area) and your fingers lightly on the temples (see illustration 17). *Hold* that position for 5 seconds.

Now, *raise* both hands simultaneously to a height of 1 to 3 inches *away* from the person's head (see illustration 18). *Hold* this position for about 60 seconds.

Then, bring your hands gently back down to the person's head again in the same original touch points (illustration 17). *Hold* for 5 seconds, and then remove them.

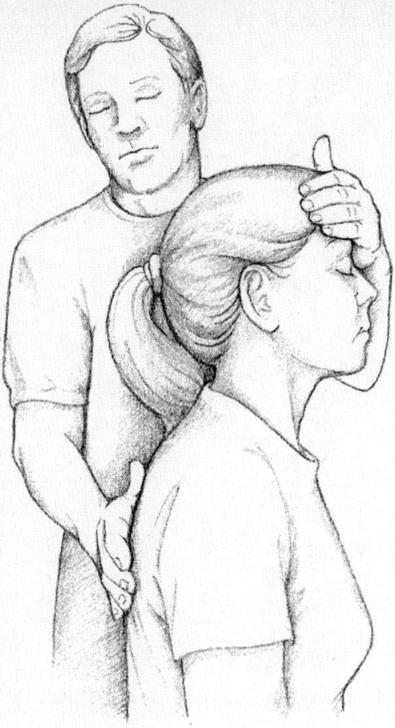

Illustration 15:

Hands ON forehead and between shoulder blades

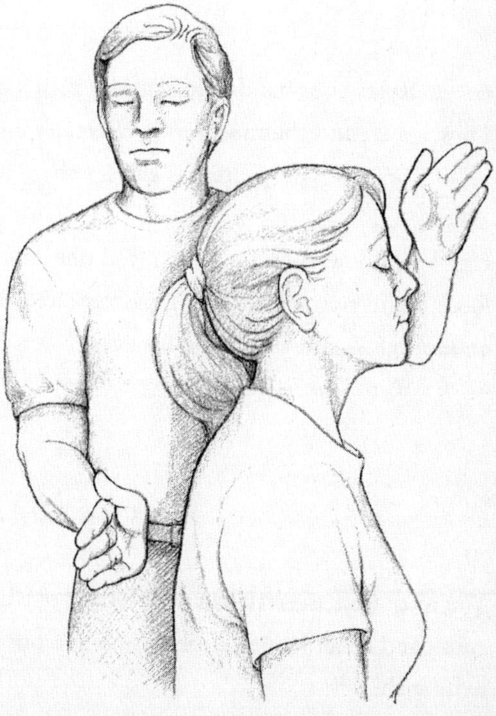

Illustration 16:

Hands 1 to 3 inches AWAY from forehead and shoulder blades

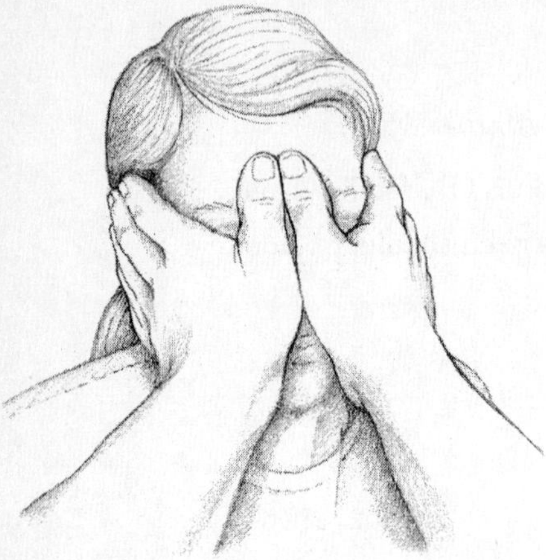

Illustration 17:

"Butterfly" ON forehead and temples

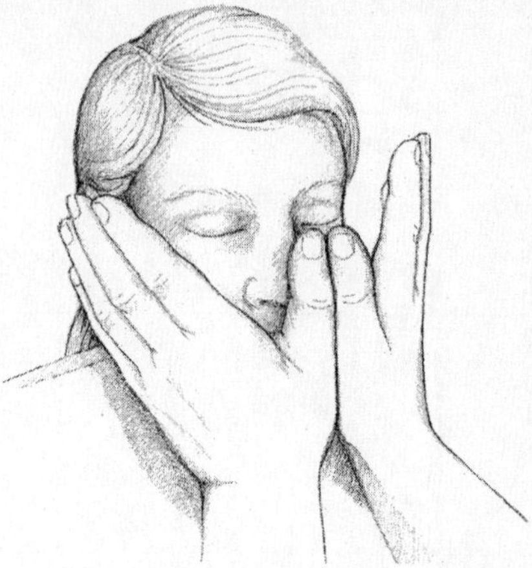

Illustration 18:

"Butterfly" 1 to 3 inches AWAY from forehead and temples

Relax your hands and arms by your sides. Tense and release them a few times, and then *shake them vigorously* for a few seconds.

Take in 3 deep breaths and let them out slowly.

STEP 8: It's now time for your loved one to *blank* his mind's screen and focus on his normal breathing pattern. Tell him to count *up* from 1 to 5 on *each exhale* and then open his eyes.

Wash your hands.

Backaches

You must first ascertain that your loved one has exhausted all medical avenues and is not having different pains from the ones she is seeking your help with.

To relieve backaches involving the lower and mid-back areas, sciatica, and the neck regions, you will need to have the person *lying face-down.* If you don't have a massage table, use a couch or bed.

Wash your hands.
Have your loved one lying face-down.
Play instrumental music, if desired.
Adjust lighting.

STEP 1: Teach and take the person through the Physical De-stressing Technique.

STEP 2: Teach and take the person through the Mental De-stressing Technique.

STEP 3: Teach and take the person through her specific self-healing visualization. The flowing band of white light should *expand* to *double its width* over the problem area. Both of you must *hold* this image for 5 seconds and then visualize healing energy waves penetrating deep into tight, knotted, and painful muscles. Mentally "see" these tight muscles unknotting, releasing, and relaxing. *Hold* this image for 5 seconds.

STEP 4: Next, tell your loved one to close her eyes and focus on her normal breathing pattern. Instruct her to mentally count *down* from 5 to 1 after *each exhale.* When she reaches 1, she should *blank* her mind's "screen" and begin her specific Self-healing Visualization Technique for her particular back ailment.

Take 3 deep breaths through your mouth and let them out slowly through your nose.

STEP 5: Stand over the person and gently place your *left* hand, fingers together, on the back of the neck area. *At the same time,* place your *right* hand

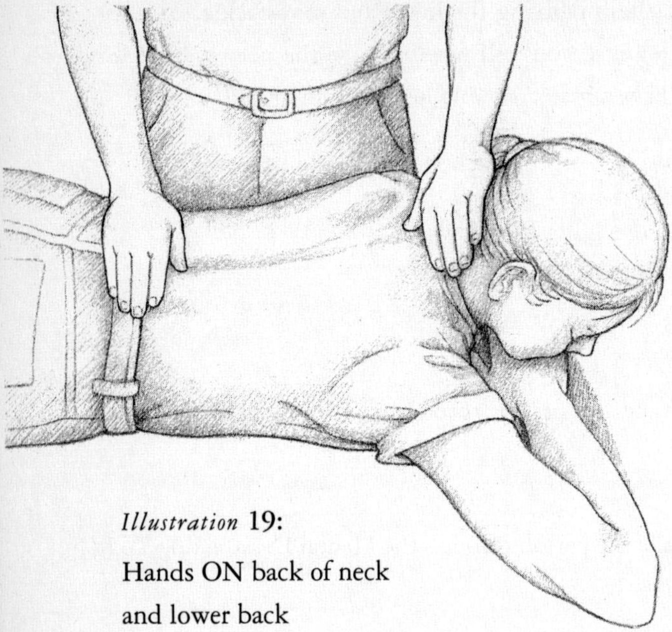

Illustration 19:
Hands ON back of neck
and lower back

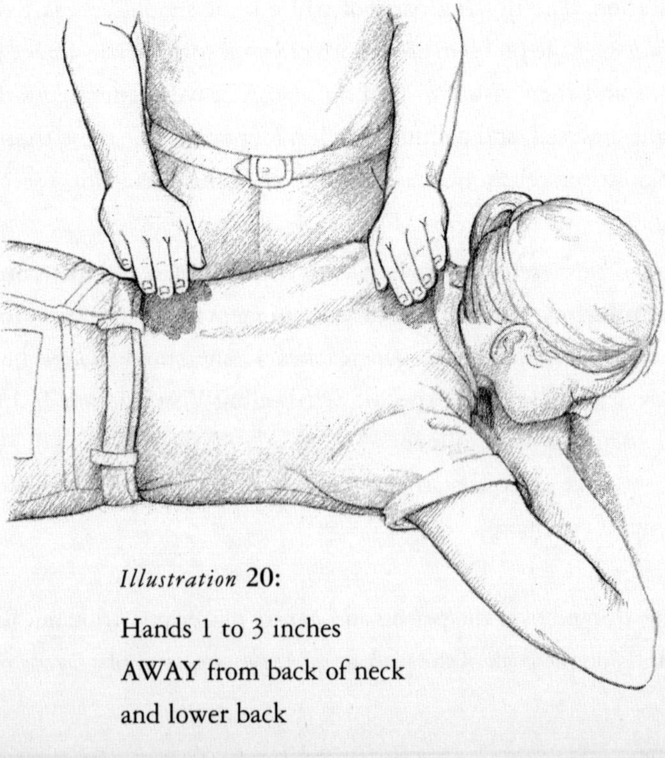

Illustration 20:
Hands 1 to 3 inches
AWAY from back of neck
and lower back

lightly on the lower-back area near the waist (see illustration 19). *Hold* your hands in these positions for 5 seconds.

Now, slowly *raise* both hands simultaneously, fingers together, to a height of 1 to 3 inches *away* from the body's surface (see illustration 20). *Hold* for about 60 seconds.

Lower both hands simultaneously to the original touch positions (illustration 19), and *hold* for 5 seconds.

Raise your hands slowly again, and put your arms by your sides as you tense, release, and relax them.

STEP 6: With hands slightly apart and fingers together, place *both* your hands lightly on the mid-back area (see illustration 21). *Hold* this position for 5 seconds.

Slowly *raise* both hands to a height of 1 to 3 inches *away* from the body (see illustration 22). *Hold* this position for at least 60 seconds.

Now, slowly lower your hands back again to the original touch-point areas (illustration 21) and *hold* for another 5 seconds.

Remove your hands and drop your arms to your sides. Tense and relax them.

STEP 7: Stand over your loved one, hands in the "butterfly" position. Gently place *both* hands *at the same time* on the mid-back area (see illustration 23) and *hold* for 5 seconds.

Now, *raise both* hands 1 to 3 inches *away* from the body (see illustration 24). *Hold* this position for about 60 seconds.

Gently lower your hands again to the same original touch points (illustration 23) and *hold* for 5 seconds.

Remove your hands and lower them to your sides. Tense and relax your hands and arms.

STEP 8: Place your *right* hand gently on the top of the person's head. *At the same time,* place your *left* hand on the back of her neck (see illustration 25). *Hold* for 5 seconds.

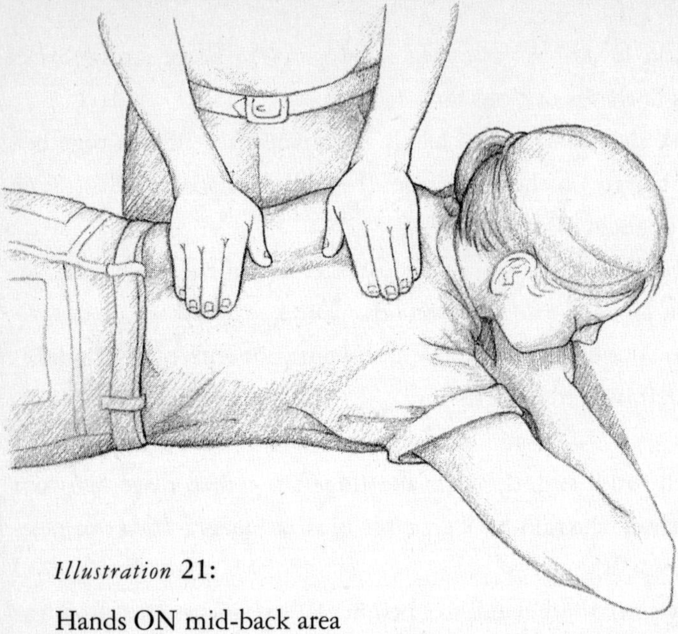

Illustration 21:

Hands ON mid-back area

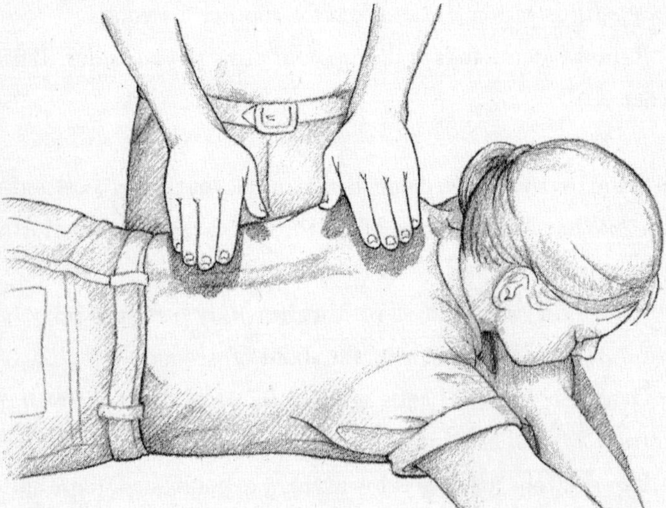

Illustration 22:

Hands 1 to 3 inches
AWAY from mid-back area

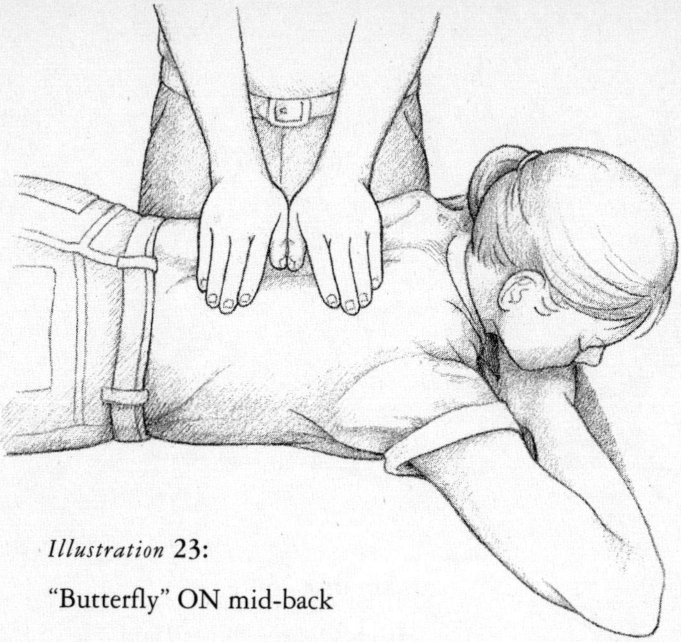

Illustration 23:

"Butterfly" ON mid-back

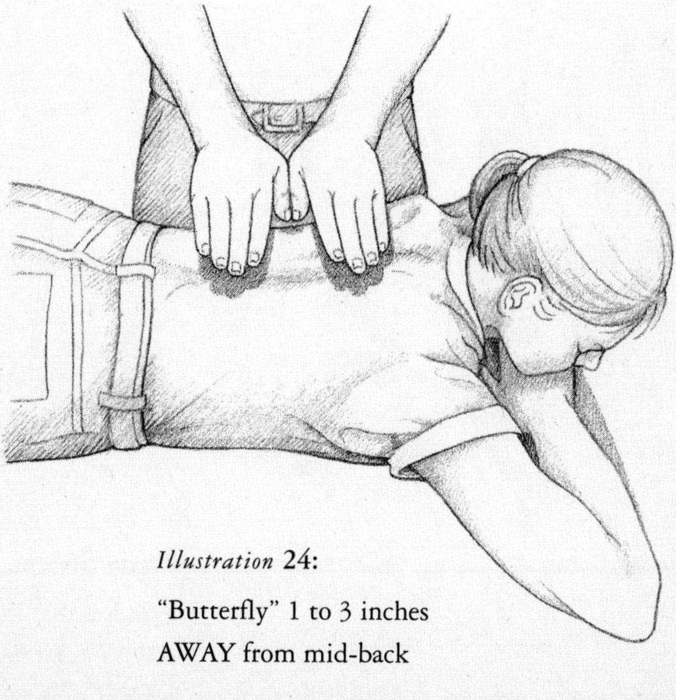

Illustration 24:

"Butterfly" 1 to 3 inches AWAY from mid-back

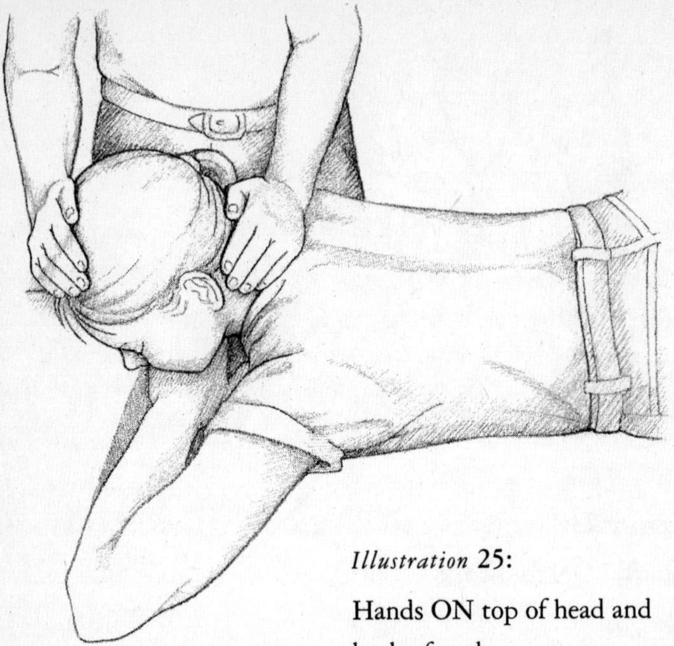

Illustration 25:

Hands ON top of head and back of neck

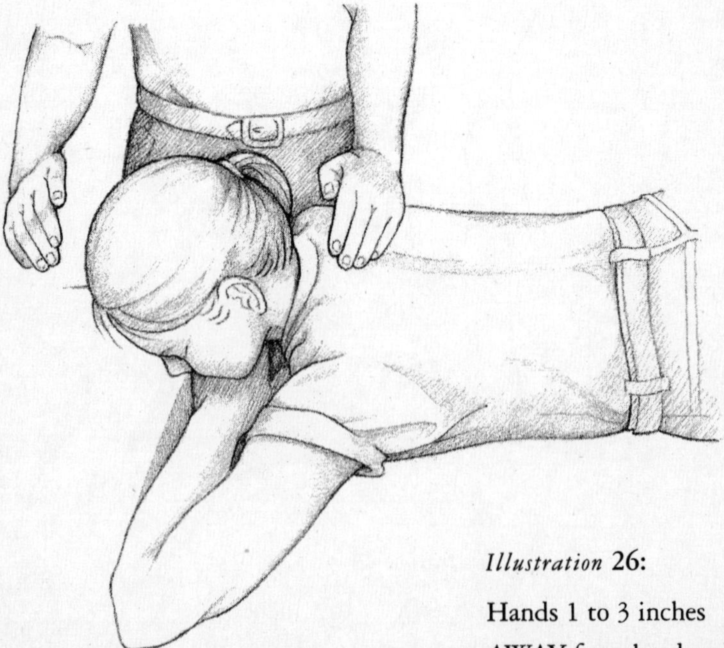

Illustration 26:

Hands 1 to 3 inches AWAY from head and back of neck

Slowly *raise* both hands to a height of 1 to 3 inches *away* from the body (see illustration 26). *Hold* for at least 60 seconds.

Gently lower your hands to the original touch points (illustration 25) and *hold* for another 5 seconds.

Remove your hands and drop them to your sides, tense and relax them. Now, *vigorously shake* both hands for a few seconds to release any accumulated energy.

Take in 3 deep breaths and exhale slowly through your nose.

STEP 9: Now, have your loved one *blank* her mind's "screen" from her specific visualization and focus on her normal breathing pattern. Instruct her to mentally count *up* from 1 to 5 on *each exhale,* and then open her eyes.

Wash your hands.

Menstrual Cramps and PMS

First, be sure that your loved one indeed has menstrual cramps and PMS symptoms, and not some other problem.

Wash your hands.
Seat your loved one in a straight-back chair.
Play instrumental music, if desired.
Adjust lighting.

STEP 1: Teach and take the person through the Physical De-stressing Technique.

STEP 2: Teach and take her through the Mental De-stressing Technique.

STEP 3: Take the person through her specific Self-healing Visualization Technique. Have her visualize healing energy waves penetrating into her lower abdomen, unknotting the painful, cramped, and tight muscles and relaxing them, freeing them of pain. Remember that it's important for you to visualize this yourself during this process.

STEP 4: Tell your loved one to close her eyes and focus on her normal breathing pattern.

Next, instruct her to mentally count *down* from 5 to 1 after *each exhale.* When she reaches 1, have her *blank* her mind's "screen." Both of you will begin the specific Self-healing Visualization Technique for menstrual cramps and PMS, mentally "seeing" the white light *expanding* into the lower abdomen.

Hold that image for 5 seconds, then visualize the healing energy waves penetrating into the cramped constricted muscles, unknotting and relaxing them.

STEP 5: Stand behind your loved one with your hands together in the "butterfly" position. Place your thumbs, which are touching each other, gently on the back of her neck. Your other fingers, all together, should surround the sides of her neck (see illustration 27). *Hold* those hand positions for 5 seconds.

Raise both your hands, still in the "butterfly" position, 1 to 3 inches *away* from the body (see illustration 28). *Hold* for at least 60 seconds.

Now, slowly lower your hands to the original touch points (illustration 27) and *hold* again for 5 seconds.

Remove your hands and drop your hands and arms by your sides. Tense and relax them.

STEP 6: Standing to the side of the person, place your *right* hand, fingers together, gently on your loved one's forehead while *at the same time* placing your *left* hand 3 inches *away* from her lower abdomen and waist area, not touching the body (see illustration 29). *Hold* this one-hand-on, one-hand-off position for 5 seconds.

Leave your *left* hand where it is (3 inches *away* from the abdomen)

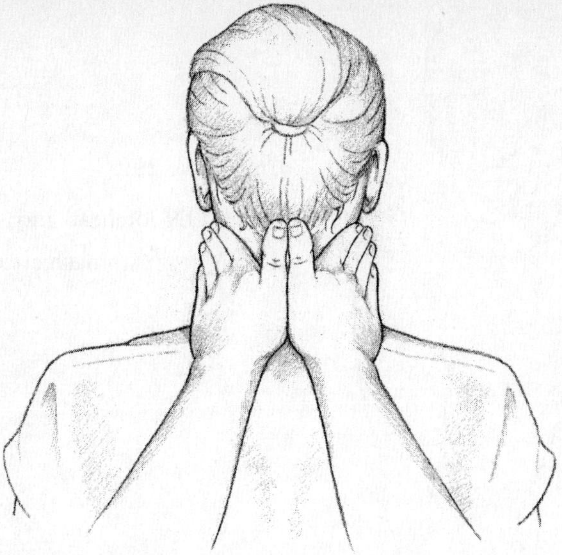

Illustration 27:

"Butterfly" ON back of neck

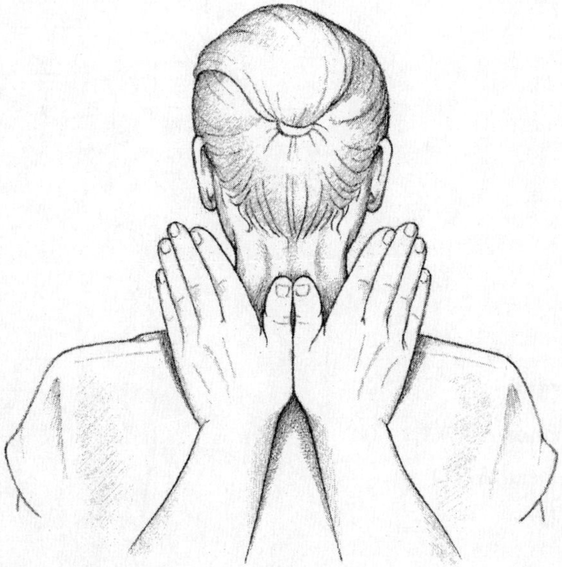

Illustration 28:

"Butterfly" 1 to 3 inches AWAY from back of neck

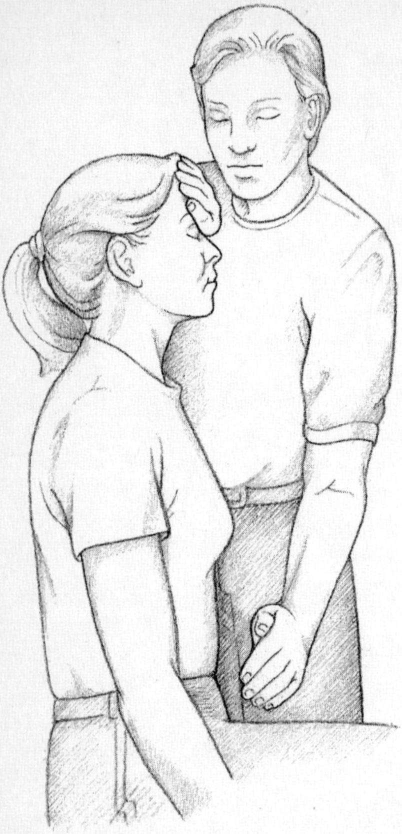

Illustration 29:

Hands ON forehead and AWAY from stomach area

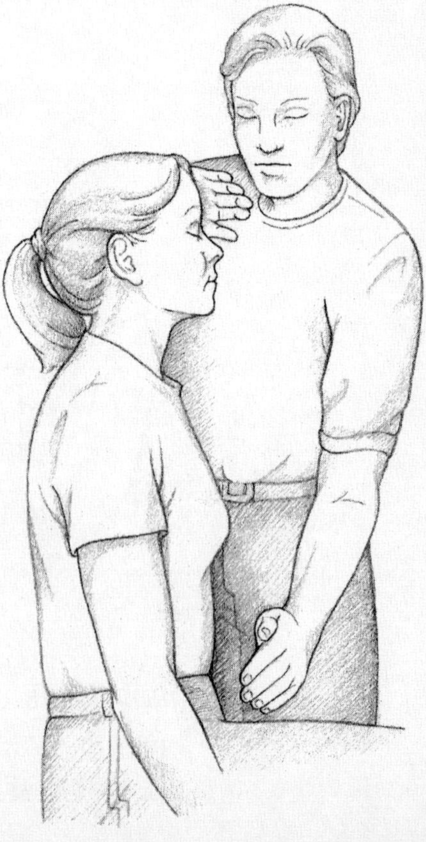

Illustration 30:

BOTH hands AWAY from forehead AND stomach area

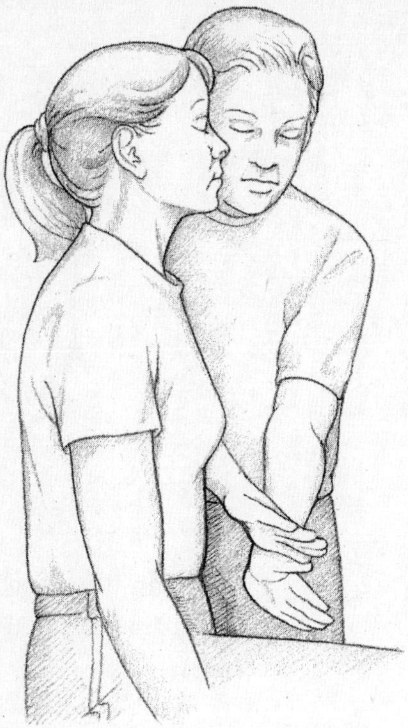

Illustration 31:
"Butterfly" 3 inches
AWAY from abdomen

and *raise* your *right* hand *only* 1 inch *away* from her forehead (see illustration 30). *Hold* both hands away from the body for at least 60 seconds.

Now, gently lower your *right* hand again to the forehead, while your *left* hand *still* maintains a 3-inch distance from the lower abdomen, in the original hand positions (illustration 29). *Hold* for another 5 seconds.

Raise both hands, drop them to your sides, and tense and relax them.

STEP 7: Form the "butterfly" position with your hands and place them 3 inches *away* from the abdomen (see illustration 31). *Hold* for 10 seconds.

Now, drop your hands to your sides, tense and relax them.

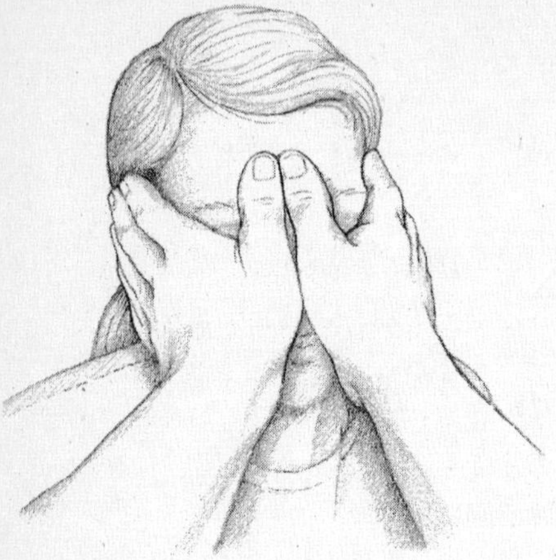

Illustration 32:

"Butterfly" ON forehead and temples

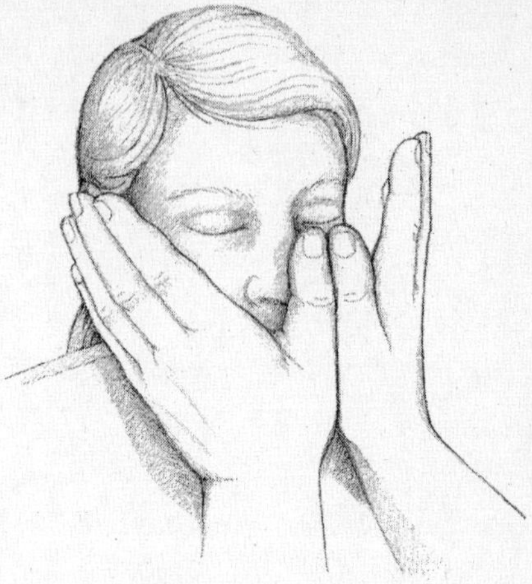

Illustration 33:

"Butterfly" 1 to 3 inches AWAY from forehead and temples

STEP 8: With your hands in the "butterfly" position, gently touch the person's "third eye" area and temples (see illustration 32). *Hold* for 5 seconds.

Raise both hands *away* from the forehead and temples 1 to 3 inches, maintaining the "butterfly" position (see illustration 33). *Hold* that position for at least 60 seconds.

Now, gently lower your hands, still in the "butterfly" position, to the original touch points (illustration 32). *Hold* again for 5 seconds.

Remove your hands and place them by your sides. Tense and relax them, then *vigorously shake both hands* for a few seconds.

Take in 3 deep breaths and exhale slowly through your nose.

STEP 9: Have your loved one *blank* her mind's "screen." Now, tell her to focus on her normal breathing pattern, mentally counting *up* from 1 to 5 on *each exhale*. When she reaches 5, tell her to open her eyes.

Wash your hands.

Reaching Out: Distant or Absent Healing

There are times when your ill loved one is either thousands of miles away or in a hospital room, connected to oxygen or a respirator, and you cannot actually be with him or touch him directly. Regardless, you can still try to stimulate the person's healing mechanism. The most simple form of distant healing is prayer, which is related to sending positive, loving, and healing thoughts to the ill person.

I believe another, even more focused, method is for you to get a picture of the person you're trying to help and, of course, find out what you can about his ailment. If it's possible, you can agree on a time when you can focus on sending your energies, while the ill person concentrates on receiving them. During this process, you can tell the person to lie down, close his eyes, and relax. It's a good idea for you to do this in a quiet, comfortable, and relaxing environment.

Before you start, I recommend that you do the physical and mental de-stressing techniques (chapter 18). The visualization you use depends on the illness. For example, when treating someone with a brain tumor, you would "see" the person's head and then a close-up of that tumor shrinking. Or, simply visualize that person well, doing the activities that used to bring him or her pleasure. If the person is paralyzed, you can "see" him or her walking or running again.

You can do this by yourself, even if you cannot communicate with the sick person. The time you devote to this practice is up to you and your schedule—you can do this from one to twenty minutes.

•

There are many other alternative therapies you can utilize besides psychic healing. In chapter 20 you'll find the answers to the most frequently asked questions about alternative healing and prevention. What does not work for one might work well for another.

20

Answers *to* Frequently Asked Questions About Alternative Healing *and* Prevention

THROUGHOUT MY TWENTY-FIVE YEARS IN THE field of alternative healing and prevention, I have received many thousands of letters, as well as queries from my own patients, about *How?*, *If?*, *Where?*, and *When?* to try psychic healing and other alternative methods. Here are the answers to some of those questions, as well as *my opinions.*

P*sychic* H*ealing*

1. *What is the difference between psychic healing, Reiki healing, and therapeutic touch?*

   Nothing. They *all* use the principles of unblocking and balancing the body's energy fields in order to stimulate another's own healing system to function properly.

2. *How is "psychic" healing different from "faith" healing?*

The term "psychic" implies using ones' "mind power" to stimulate another person's healing, whereas "faith" healing uses *your belief* in God, Jesus, or other religious principles. As far as I'm concerned, it's not the *means* but the *end results* that count, so utilize whatever method is most comfortable for you.

3. *When should I go to a psychic healer?*

First and foremost, go only when medical science has done all it can for you. I suggest going to a psychic healer if you were not as successful at self-healing as you would have liked or if other alternative therapies have not been effective.

4. *How long should I see a psychic healer?*

I suggest that you give this therapy, as well as any other alternative treatment, a fair chance—approximately 3 to 5 sessions over a period of a month—to see if you have any improvements. Once you begin to see positive change, continue with the practitioner for as long as it is helpful and you keep experiencing progress.

5. *Do I have to "believe" to be healed?*

Not in my experience, for many skeptical people that did not believe in psychic healing *still* received help from my ministrations. However, I found also that the more close-minded and resistant you are, the longer it may take for you to receive the beneficial results you're seeking.

6. *What is the best attitude for me to have in order to be the most receptive to my healer?*

I suggest a positive, open-minded approach. The number-one prerequisite is that you *believe* in *yourself* and that you *will* get better. This conviction needs to be *unshakable,* regardless of the healing catalyst you employ.

7. *How do I persuade a loved one or friend to try laying-on-of-hands healing?*
First, you can have your loved one speak with someone who *has benefited* from this therapy. Or, you can offer the person information regarding the healer's qualifications. It would be very helpful for you to find any published articles or a book about the healer's work, so that your loved one can read about the practitioner him- or herself. It's also possible that any medical doctors who refer their own patients to that healer would be happy to speak with your loved one.

8. *Will my medical doctor help me find a psychic healer?*
Twenty-five years ago, I would have said, "Never," but today, more and more physicians are embracing psychic healing and other alternative therapies as complementary or adjunctive therapies to be employed when medical science has not been effective. *Do not* be intimidated to ask your doctor if you might fall into that category—he/she may very well have heard about, or personally know, a psychic healer to recommend. If not, ask your friends, family, or associates if their own doctors ever have recommended a laying-on-of-hands healer. If you still have no luck, then you need to do some research at your local library or bookstore.

9. *If someone has a "gift" for healing with the hands, why should they charge for this service? Is there a guarantee that it will help me?*
Anyone who offers a specialized service has the right to be paid for his or her time and expertise. A doctor charges his or her fee whether or not you are helped, so why not an alternative therapist? There are *no guarantees* that you will be healed in *any* field of alternative healing *or* medical science.

10. *When I begin to see a psychic healer, can I stop seeing my medical doctor?*
No. It is *important* to *continue* to see your physician so he/she can monitor and document your progress with your psychic healer or whatever alternative therapy you want to try. You will greatly ben-

efit from a better working relationship between the alternative healer and the medical doctor.

11. *If I break my arm, can I go just to my psychic healer?*
No. Here's the perfect situation that a traditional Western medical doctor can well handle—X rays, a cast, etc. A break in a bone that is not set properly can give you only more problems in the future. Psychic healing is *not* an alternative to traditional Western medicine. Each has its proper place and time.

12. *Can psychic healing help severe abdominal pains?*
When you have extreme pains *anywhere* in your body, immediately go to your medical doctor or to a hospital emergency room—you might have appendicitis or some other serious problem that needs prompt medical attention. Otherwise, you are *risking your life*!

13. *What can I do during the treatment to be more responsive to my psychic healer?*
Every psychic healer or alternative practitioner should have his or her own methods for helping patients relax and calm their minds and bodies. If you find yourself undergoing a therapy that does not, I recommend you familiarize yourself with my physical and mental de-stressing techniques (see chapter 18).

14. *Is Shiatsu a form of psychic healing?*
It is similar *only* to the point that both methods attempt to balance and unblock the energy fields in the body. But practitioners of shiatsu, which is based on traditional Oriental principles, *do* use strong, deep-finger *pressure and manipulation* at predetermined points on the body, and sometimes this can be very painful.

Psychic healing uses no pressure or manipulation, only light touching and energy-field work, 1 to 3 inches above the body. Undergoing psychic healing is *not* supposed to be a painful process. If it is, find another psychic healer! The one you are seeing might be an inexperienced practitioner.

15. *Will pursuing a variety of alternative therapies at the same time help me get better faster?*
Not at all, and I definitely would *not* recommend doing this. I believe you need to give each therapy the exclusive opportunity to help you. Otherwise, confusion can reign in your mind and body. As the saying goes, "Too many cooks *can* spoil the broth." And, if you *do* get well, you won't know what helped you and what didn't.

I really feel it would be much more effective for you to engage in *one alternative therapy at a time.* Give each therapy a month to six weeks, once a week, to see if you are improving. Remember: More is not better!

16. *Can alternative therapies conflict with one another?*
I believe they can, because I've had numerous cases in which the ill person gained negative results. One case in particular involved a young woman with interstitial cystitis, a painful bladder problem. In the three months we worked together, she responded well to my ministrations, her symptoms disappeared, and she went into remission. The following month, when she came back for a maintenance treatment, she asked if she could also try an acupuncturist for a different minor problem. Not wanting to stand in her way, I agreed.

Somehow, in one single session, the acupuncture treatment managed to *undo* all the positive effects I was able to stimulate in three months, and all her painful bladder symptoms returned in full force.

That experience really taught me a lesson: With few exceptions, *do not mix therapies*! In the first half of my healing career, I allowed my patients to do whatever they wanted. Even though many still responded to my efforts, there is no question in my mind that in later years, when I *did* restrict them from combining therapies, they responded to my treatments *much* more quickly.

17. *What is this "healing energy" made of? Does the energy emanating from the psychic healer's hands have anything to do with electromagnetism?*
In my experience, I have found that healing energy can *affect* not only electromagnetic fields, but also electrostatic fields and biological and physical mechanisms. Electromagnetism might play a small role in the equation of what makes up this force field, but I believe, based on previous research I've conducted, that it does not play a major role in its composition. This energy still is being studied today so we can understand how it can affect the body, but scientists have not figured out what it's really made of. Hopefully, in the years to come, with more diligent research, we might finally uncover the essence of healing energy. I just hope that this energy is not as elusive as love, which I feel is the most important ingredient in this healing recipe.

18. *I have cancer and have undergone all the appropriate medical treatments, but with no success. Recently, I tried a laying-on-of-hands healer, but it's been several weeks and I'm not improving yet. I'm becoming very discouraged. Should I give up hope?*
Never! First of all, a few weeks with *any* alternative healer is not a long time, especially if you like the practitioner and he/she has a gentle touch and manner. You have to be more patient and allow time for the healing to take place, especially with cancer. I have found it frequently takes a little longer to see results when the patient has a serious illness. However, if after another few weeks of treatment you still don't feel you're making any headway, then I would seek out another laying-on-of-hands healer or try another alternative healing therapy.

Remember: Everyone is different. What works for one might not work for another. If one psychic healer does not help you, do not hesitate to search out a different one. Do NOT give up hope! Hope catalysts the will to live, and it comes in many forms, so never give up. Just try another healer and be persevering—you still could get your *miracle*!

19. *What is psychic surgery? Do you recommend it?*

I know of several medical doctors and paranormal investigators who have researched psychic surgery, which is commonly practiced in the Philippines. Various well-documented films have showcased these exhibitions. Typically, this process involves an alleged "psychic surgeon" laying the patient out on a table, using unadorned hands and fingers as "knives," and supposedly creating an "opening" in a patient's body, removing diseased matter and leaving behind a trail of blood and tissue, but no scar. In the films, these practitioners were diligent in disposing of this material, but a few times an enterprising investigator was able to retrieve a well-hidden portion from the garbage. It is discouraging to me that not once did a piece of tissue taken from a psychic surgeon's procedure ever turn out to be diseased tissue from that same patient.

I remember one particular film documented that a piece of material removed from someone was stolen immediately after the "surgical" procedure, and it turned out to be a pregnant woman's mammary tissue. Now, you might think, "Well, that's proof," except the patient was a man. The journalist learned that this tissue was easily available and obtainable from most hospital disposal areas. Some psychic surgeons were caught on film palming animal guts and blood and using a clever sleight-of-hand maneuver—kneading the fatty areas of the stomach or other parts of the body to make the patient and observers think they were seeing a real incision in the body cavity and diseased tissue removed. As far as I am concerned, people should stay far away from this unsterile and questionable therapy.

Other Alternative Healing Therapies

20. *What is "crystal" healing, and how effective is it?*

In this form of therapy, precious stones, gems, and natural crystals that emit certain healing "vibrations" are worn by or placed on the body of the ill person. In all of my experiences, I have yet to see any major clinical improvement effected by crystal healing. If *I* had a serious health problem, I would not put all my hope into crystal healing alone. If you still want to try it, I would suggest you use it as an *adjunctive* therapy to *another* alternative method that has been proven to be effective in helping your health condition.

I believe more research needs to be conducted into the efficacy of crystal healing and its possible benefits. If your health problem has not responded to medical treatment or numerous alternative therapies, then by all means give crystal healing, performed by an experienced practitioner, a try. It can't hurt you.

21. *My doctors tell me I'm going to die from cancer within a few months. I am in the process of trying an alternative therapy, but, at this point, will having a "positive" or "hopeful" outlook really make a difference in whether or not I respond?*

Absolutely! If there is one word that is essential in the fight for life from cancer, it's "attitude." It could certainly mean the difference between life and death. Of course, medical science, with its usually preset prognoses on how long a person will live with whatever cancer he or she has, does *not* help induce a positive attitude for the patient. If anything, it depresses and *robs* the patient of *hope,* so he or she starts out on an uneven emotional playing field.

A psychiatrist I worked with in New York City in the early years, who had observed and documented many of my healing sessions with his own patients, is one of many sad examples.

Somehow, I never thought that with all of his psychological perceptions, psychiatric training, and comprehension, he would become a *victim* himself. He was diagnosed with chronic lymphatic leukemia, but he was the picture of health. He experienced no pain and continued to work with his usual zest for life, helping others.

But *the day after his prognosis* of "three months to live," he changed completely. He was deflated, depressed, and suddenly took on a sickly appearance. It seemed that he *believed* the prognosis and lost his will to live. He fulfilled his doctor's prophecy and died three months later, almost to the day.

This loss, among others, burned into my mind the importance of having a *positive attitude*—not only when you're battling cancer, but with *any* health problem. I am convinced that a determined and optimistic demeanor can help change the course of cancer or any disease. I know it can make an amazing difference between giving up and believing a doctor's dire predictions, or fighting for your life. I have seen people stricken with terrible diseases who had very optimistic and hopeful points of view—"No way, doctor! Not me! I'm going to fight this disease all the way down the line!"—and *many of them* did just that! They did not allow the doctors' often-mistaken time-line prognoses to discourage them and stamp out their hope—they propelled themselves toward researching alternative therapies that, in many cases, proved helpful or even life-saving. Also, many did self-help techniques to stimulate their own healing systems and sense of well-being.

22. *Are the current diagnostic procedures in alternative therapies as accurate as the most recent medical technologies?*

Go to your medical doctor to be diagnosed—not to *any* alternative therapist. Most alternative "diagnosticians" are not accurate, are often misleading, and can send many ill people on unnecessary wild-goose chases, wasting their precious time by not offering *proper* diagnoses and treatments.

For instance, there are *psychics* who diagnose. I feel they are indirectly and unintentionally projecting negative or incorrect images into people's minds that might actually be harmful. Our minds are fertile, powerful, and creative instruments, so if some "psychic" tells a client that he or she has a liver condition, and the person does *not*—who knows? Maybe this person will "mentally" create it!

My advice to all psychics, unless you are being monitored and documented by a medical doctor, *do not* give your clients your opinion or "vibes," negative *or* positive, pertaining to their health.

There are many alternative therapies that "diagnose" in a nebulous manner. In my experience, I have found that most traditional Oriental practitioners of acupuncture, shiatsu, qi gong, etc., do not give as accurate or complete a diagnostic picture as traditional Western doctors. The same goes for iridology (diagnosing through the eyes), reflexology, homeopathy, osteopathy, hair analysis, etc.

I also especially suggest you avoid any nutritionist or chiropracter that uses a *machine* or *computer* to diagnose. I've *never* seen a person properly diagnosed in this manner, nor a controlled research study proving that *any* alternative therapist can diagnose with the same accuracy as traditional Western physicians.

I am *not* saying that these alternative therapies don't work. I *am* saying that practitioners of those therapies should avoid *diagnosing* and stick to being healing catalysts.

23. *I'm taking Chinese herbs and some homeopathic remedies. Are they safe?*
I advise you to proceed with caution. A recent study in Britain showed that twenty-one people were poisoned and two died from ingesting certain Chinese herbs. I personally don't believe that anyone should take *any* alternative health substance that has not been properly studied, approved, regulated, and sanctioned by the Food and Drug Administration, the National Institutes of Health, or other countries' health-governing organizations.

The homeopath diagnoses the patient, then presents a remedy.

Homeopathic remedies are based on the theory that "like treats like," and supposedly act as a catalyst, jump-starting the body to heal itself.

However, I believe this alternative therapy really needs more medical and scientifically controlled studies to determine its possible benefits. Published studies have reported that a number of people who have taken certain homeopathic substances have complained of negative side effects, so you need to be cautious before trying any therapy in which you have to eat or swallow anything!

Unfortunately, I've had several occasions in which people sought my help because they had taken Chinese herbs or homeopathic remedies that gave them adverse effects. If you are inclined to utilize these substances, I would advise you to research and network to get dependable information on which ones to avoid and which are reportedly safe.

24. *Will my health insurance pay for alternative therapies?*

Call your insurance representative and carefully read your policy. Every day, more alternative therapies are being covered in part or fully through insurance, and certain companies have separate riders that do include coverage of various alternative options. Many of the insurance companies in countries such as Great Britain, the Netherlands and other European and Asian countries are already including alternative treatments in their coverage. The United States is moving at a little slower pace, but new options are being added to the growing list of choices covered by insurance, which once cast a jaundiced eye toward anything other than traditional Western medical treatments.

25. *Is reflexology like the laying on of hands?*

Reflexology has its roots in traditional Chinese pressure methods and is similar to psychic healing in that both therapies try to balance and unblock the energy's pathways around the body to stimulate the patient's own healing mechanism. The main difference is that reflexologists apply the pressure mainly to the soles of the feet. I think it can be very relaxing, excellent for the circulation, and even has its own self-help aspects.

26. *I'm used to having full-body deep massages, and it really helps relax me. Recently, I've been diagnosed with bone cancer in my rib cage and spine. Is it still safe to have them?*

I would *not* suggest undergoing *any* deep pressing or manipulating therapies such as acupressure, shiatsu, chiropractics, or even deep massage if you have diseased or brittle bones caused by cancer, rheumatoid or osteoarthritis, osteoporosis, or any similar condition. For years I've treated people with these problems whose situations were worsened by pain or even bone fractures caused by overzealous body workers.

One case in point was Frank Zappa, whom I treated for prostate cancer and bone metastasis. One day, Frank told me he was beginning to see a massage therapist. According to what he described, the therapist used a vigorous form of deep massage. After a few days, Frank said he felt very sore—his whole body hurt.

Because Frank had lesions and fragility in his bones, I felt that strong massage, pressure, or manipulation could actually be detrimental to his condition, and I persuaded him to discontinue it. He stopped the massages and soon felt much better.

This experience made me realize also that if you are responding well to an alternative therapy, *don't mess with what's working*! Don't add additional therapies, thinking you'll get well faster. I've found it doesn't work that way and, in fact, combined therapies could create negative results for the patient.

27. *I've already had surgery for breast cancer and completed my chemotherapy regimen. After losing thirty pounds, I'm down to skin and bones. Now my*

friend is suggesting I go to her macrobiotic dietician. I'll try anything to get well. What do you think?

I think it would be like *committing suicide*! An extreme macrobiotic diet with your specific condition will only make you lose even more weight, creating a further strain on your body. Additionally, it will compromise your already battered and depressed immune system.

I feel that in the position you're in, you do not want to lose weight, but *gain* weight through a good *balanced nutritional* regimen, so your body's own healing system will work optimally. Macrobiotic diets discourage you from eating animal foods, sugar, and meat, and severely restrict and limit your intake of fluids. This can be very dangerous, for the body requires large quantities of liquids for proper metabolism. When you're most in need of vitamins and minerals, this diet proves deficient.

You need to work with a nutritional therapist who will encourage you to *gain* and not lose weight. You *need* the *strength to fight*!

28. *I have stomach cancer, and my doctors have given up on me. I was referred to an immunotherapy practitioner in Mexico. Do you think this will help my problem?*

I personally do not believe in this particular treatment, for I have seen too many patients have terrible experiences with it.

A well-known comedian's wife recommended me to her brother, who had abdominal cancer. He was in his early thirties, and right before seeing me, he had been in a clinic in Mexico for a form of chemical immunotherapy, which is illegal in the United States. He told me he had been to this clinic several times, and since he began this highly toxic treatment, his stomach and colon tumors had suddenly grown.

I had the opportunity to work with him for only about a week, but he still reported feeling better and stronger since this whole downward spiral had begun. So I was surprised when he said he was going back to Mexico to question the clinicians about this new active growth of his cancer.

When he went back down there, he instead underwent further treatments. He never made it back from Mexico alive.

His case was not an isolated one—I have heard from a disturbing number of patients about ill family members who were administered non-FDA-approved drugs in the Bahamas, as well as in Mexico, and came back home, but in pine boxes. I believe there are plenty of other effective and much safer alternative therapies. Stay away from unapproved alternative immunological treatments!

29. *Can I combine color therapy with psychic healing to help my rheumatoid arthritis?*

Colors of the spectrum are used to help stimulate and balance our physical, emotional, and spiritual bodies. Tinted lights and colors are the subtle tools of the color therapist. The color of water, tinted natural oils, colors in your home, and even the hues of your clothing all are instruments that the therapist teaches you to use more efficiently in your daily life.

I believe this therapy is definitely a complementary one, to be used at the same time with other alternative healing therapies. Do not use it alone if you have any type of serious health problem.

30. *What is aroma therapy massage? What problems can it help?*

Aroma therapists *massage* into your skin different essential plant aromatic oils that are supposed to help certain *minor* problems such as acne, backaches, headaches, constipation, and muscle aches.

It can be a very relaxing, soothing, and pampering experience if the massage is not too deep or painful. It is another good complementary therapy to other alternative techniques.

31. *I've been told that self-hypnosis is helpful and combines well with other healing therapies. Is this true?*

Yes. Self-hypnosis is certainly a useful self-help and complementary method. This on-command, self-inducing relaxant definitely has helped people respond better to my ministrations as well as to other alternative therapies.

Self-hypnosis is very helpful also when learning, practicing, and comprehending self-help visualizations. Many people seem to have fewer problems understanding and implementing these techniques when they have had some training in self-hypnosis. Of course, the hypnotherapist that teaches you should come well recommended.

32. *A friend of mine has cancer, and now he sleeps on a bed filled with large magnets. He insists it's the same energy as from an energy healer's hands. Is he right?*

Definitely not! In fact, I recently saw a patient with sarcoma lung cancer who went to a therapist in Canada. The therapist put him in a state-of-the-art CT scan–like machine that produced tremendously powerful magnetic fields. The patient underwent this treatment for four days. He told me that within a couple of weeks, his lung lesions grew to almost three times their sizes!

This horror story was only one of the many I've heard about ill people sleeping on magnetic beds or wearing magnets on their bodies. There has not been enough, if any, proper research conducted on the side effects of these devices. My opinion: Stay away!

Prevention

33. *Various forms of cancer run throughout my family. Is there anything I can do to help prevent myself from becoming another statistic?*

It has become common knowledge that *stress,* and especially our *reactions* to it, can harm and inhibit our bodies' immune and healing systems. I believe that in addition to practicing mental and physical stress-reducing, preventative, self-healing techniques, you need to *change* your *approach* to how you *do* respond to strain and adversity in your life.

Try to maintain a *positive attitude.* Negative thinking creates stress, and stress can inflame and even create illness. You need to be in more control over *what* you think and *how* you react. You need *not* be a casualty of your genetic situation or of negative thoughts—*deflect* them with a positive and hopeful attitude and, again, do preventative self-help exercises. Just because you may be predisposed to certain illnesses doesn't automatically mean you will get them or that you won't be able to conquer them.

34. *How can I protect myself from catching colds, flus, and possibly worse in public places?*

It all begins with awareness. Before you go out, place a mental protective shield of white light and positivity around yourself. When you come home from being outdoors, wash your hands immediately with soap and hot water for at least twelve seconds. When Rochelle and I are in a grocery store and we hear someone sneeze, as if on cue, the two of us turn around and avoid the contamination. Yes, germs travel fast and over a wide expanse, however, why, knowingly, stroll through an area with a fresh onslaught of active and live airborne germs? Wash your hands as often as you go out. I believe you cannot be too obsessive about washing your hands upon returning home.

When a friend or relative has a cold or flu, if you can possibly avoid contact with him, do so. If it's unavoidable, wear a germ mask, don't drink from his glass or eat from his plate or utensils, and don't kiss him! Again, wash your hands frequently and put up your mental protective shield. If you are particularly susceptible to flu, avoid public places during flu season as much as possible.

It would also be wise for you to avoid sitting in a doctor's office too long—waiting rooms are prime breeding grounds for all sorts of contagious germs. The dentist's office also is a tremendous source of germs. Be certain your dentist uses the most up-to-date sterilization techniques on the instruments. Don't be afraid to ask the dentist if he utilizes an autoclave, a high-powered sterilizing and disinfecting machine, on *all* his instruments *as well as their handles* before each patient. The studies on transference of diseases through lack of proper sterilization in the dentist's office are frightening.

35. *Sometimes I come home from a public place feeling completely drained. Is the problem with me or others? Can I prevent this from happening?*

Public places are natural energy drainers. I really don't believe there are "psychic vampires" walking around, saying to themselves, "Now, whose energy can I suck today?" However, I do believe that regular people can "unconsciously" drain from one another.

The same can happen in your home, or over the telephone. How many times do you get off the phone with a friend who's just shared his or her problems with you and you're exhausted?

Yes, you can prevent this. Before going out or even at home or on the telephone, you should create a protective "mental shield" that surrounds and protects you from being drained—and it's important that you remind yourself to *maintain* your shield. This attitude and process works. Give it a try, and maybe it will work for you.

36. *I am basically a happy, healthy, and optimistic middle-aged woman with no known genetic predispositions. Do you have any ideas on how I can stay healthy?*

I would suggest regular mild exercise, like light walking or swimming. I would also do meditation, de-stressing techniques, and preventative self-help exercises. You need only ten minutes each day to maintain your energy level and keep your immunity well boosted. Eat a low-fat diet, include several servings each of fruits and vegetables daily, and drink lots of water.

37. *I once read an article that laughter is the best medicine of all. Do you think this is true?*

This is very true, indeed, and there is clinical proof. Recent research has shown that laughter spontaneously stimulates the body's production of endorphins (natural relaxant and pain-reliever), as well as the inherent antidepressants serotonin and dopamine, which are especially good for the lungs and bronchial tracts. They also stimulate the immune system.

So watch sitcoms and stand-up comics, rent comedy films, and read books that tickle your funny bone.

38. *Can placebos really help?*

It's been proven that placebos can indeed stimulate the same natural healing substances in the brain as do medicines and alternative therapies. In fact, I feel doctors and hospitals should integrate a placebo program when all else fails. For too many years, the placebo has been given a backseat in the health-care industry. It's time to bring placebos to the forefront of the newly paved alternative road to better health.

39. *Do you believe it's important that there is cooperation between my medical doctor and my alternative healer?*

In order for unconventional healing methods to make their mark in the mainstream, I do believe better cooperation needs to be firmly established between the medical/scientific communities and the nontraditional practitioners. It's not up to the doctors only to take the first step—it's also the responsibility of holistic healers to stimulate interest and curiosity in their specific supplemental therapies through their successful case histories. There are still far too many doctors ignoring the possible benefits of alternative therapies, and there are too many alternative therapists who don't bother to document their work and garner the support of the medical establishment.

I also feel it would be inappropriate for medical doctors to simply refer a patient to any therapist without monitoring the practitioner and the patient's progress from the onset and documenting its efficacy. It will take medical and scientific documentation to persuade the majority of doctors that alternative healing methods can play a viable role in the health-care system.

During this process, I feel these same physicians will also uncover flawed, dangerous, and even fraudulent therapies, as well as those that are clinically helpful. The doctors will then be in a better position to both caution and enlighten the public.

40. *I have terminal cancer. My doctor said there is no hope and sent me home to die. Now what?*

When medical doctors give up on people, they must not take away the patients' last glimmers of hope. They need to support and not judge the patients in their quests to find that hope.

As nutritional food, exercise, and a positive attitude all are essential components for a healthy life, so is hope. Hope fuels the will to live, and what could possibly be more essential than that? Doctors should not ignore offering hope to their seriously ill or terminal patients. I understand their concern that patients will receive "false hope," but that's actually a contradiction of terms. The doctors don't want to raise their patients' expectations or disappoint them. However, without hope, there are *no* expectations!

Your physician should not deny you the hope that alternative therapy can bring you, as long as you continue to see your medical doctors and have your progress properly monitored. I would recommend you speak with your friends and other doctors and be referred to an alternative healer.

Patients want honesty from their physicians, but they also crave optimism and yearn for something else to try. When the doctors' attitudes and perspectives change, then their patients will be less frightened and intimidated and will, at the very least, be left with a glimmer of hope—and sometimes that is all it takes!

•

All of these questions have been answered with *my* opinions, and my responses are based on my experience and research.

It would be prudent for anyone who is looking for an alternative therapy to research and seek his or her *own* answers about any alternative health path they wish to travel. You are the one who has to be completely comfortable and satisfied with the answers to your questions, because *you* are the one who will undergo the treatment. Remember: *You are in the driver's seat! Don't ever give up hope!*

Epilogue

IN MY WILDEST DREAMS I NEVER THOUGHT THIS is what my life would become. It is certainly not what I had planned, but I know now that I have been blessed rather than cursed. I hope I have used my gifts to the best of my ability and for the highest good.

If I have accomplished anything at all, I hope it was to make laying-on-of-hands energy healing less dubious, more palatable. I hope also that by documenting my case histories and subjecting myself to scientific and medical investigations, I have helped make this alternative approach more credible and acceptable, and have made people *think.*

To the people I have touched, I thank you for letting me into a part of your lives, for it has made me a better person. *I* have learned from *you.* If you have walked away with something that has made a difference in your lives, attitudes, or health, then I am truly grateful.

Are there others out there like me? If there are, let my story be a signpost for you. For those who are still searching to find out who they are or what they might become, let me be a lesson. You never can guess what unexpected paths your life might take.

It has been an extraordinary life. My unusual career has been a long, arduous journey the past twenty-five years, full of never-ending struggles, unseen pitfalls, disappointments, and monumental victories. When I think back on my life to this point, I am left with a tremendous sense of well-being and peace of mind because of all the lessons I have learned, the paths I have crossed, and the lives I have touched. And the most important lesson of all: We all need a touch of hope.

Afterword

John M. Kmetz, Ph.D.

THE PRECEDING PAGES HAVE BEEN AN ACCOUNT of Dean Kraft's capacity to affect natural and physical systems in an unusual way. The majority of the work deals with Dean Kraft's gift as a healer. Numerous examples have been given of his power to somehow channel his energy to an affected person to effect a cure. It is noteworthy not only that he has healed people suffering from a variety of diseases, but that many of these people have been referred to him by their physicians.

The case histories of these people, both before and after treatment by Mr. Kraft, are substantive proof that he can somehow accelerate the normal healing process of the body, even in the case of cancer. Cases of spontaneous cancer remission do occur, which imply that the body has the ability to initiate cancer regression. However, our knowledge about the exact causes of cancer is far from complete, and we know even less about the process of spontaneous remission.

In an attempt to understand his ability, Dean Kraft has taken part in a number of interesting scientific experiments at respected research institutions, and has demonstrated both his ability to influence physical systems and his ability to change another person's physiological functions by a "laying on of hands." At Lawrence Livermore Laboratories in California, he was able to cause cancer cells to detach and float free from the surface on which they were growing.

The cell study was subsequently repeated at Science Unlimited Research Foundation in San Antonio, Texas, with the same results. I was at that time director of SURF and supervised the experiments. Dean Kraft consistently caused cancer cells to detach from their growing surface and float free in the culture medium, indicating that they were destroyed. Even though the results of these tests were exciting, they gave no clues concerning the nature of the energy form emanating from Dean Kraft.

This has been the story of an individual's attempts to understand not only the changes that have occurred in his life, but also to learn whether or not his healing ability can be characterized scientifically. It points to the need for more research in this area. For example, can we characterize the nature of the interaction between the healer and a patient? Can we characterize the energy involved? And finally, can individuals be trained to exhibit this ability? Only future research will give us the answers.

JOHN M. KMETZ